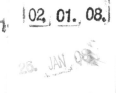

D0505041

Eat You

Rosemary Conley is the UK's most successful diet and fitness expert and has sold over 5 million books and 3 million videos on the subject. Together with her husband, Mike Rimmington, Rosemary runs three companies: Rosemary Conley Diet and Fitness Clubs Ltd, which operates a national network of almost 2,000 classes weekly; Quorn House Publishing Ltd, which publishes Rosemary Conley's Diet & Fitness magazine with a circulation of over 20,000; and Rosemary Conley Enterprises.

Dean Simpole-Clarke is one of Britain's most prominent young cooks. A rising television chef with many credits to his name, Dean runs a catering company with his wife, Julie, from their delicatessen, Simpole Clarke, in Stamford, where the emphasis is on organic foods. Dean has worked with Rosemary in creating recipes for her highly acclaimed *Red Wine Diet*, *Low Fat Cookbook* and *Low Fat Cookbook Two*. In addition, Dean continues to work with Rosemary on her various television cookery programmes.

For details of your nearest Rosemary Conley

700028020743

call 01 509 620 222

To subscribe to Rosemary Conley Diet & Fitness magazine,
call 01 509 620 444

www.rosemary-conley.co.uk

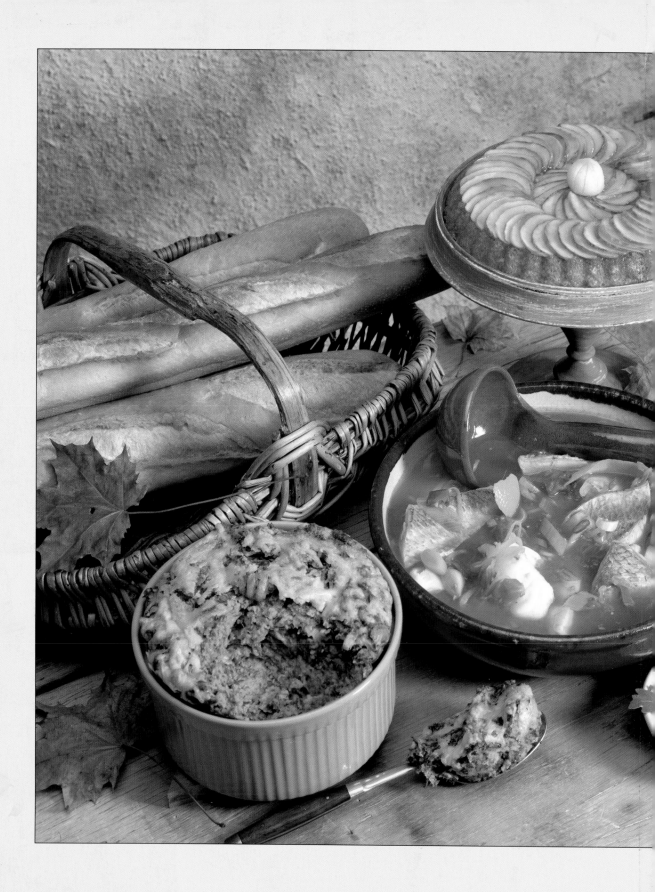

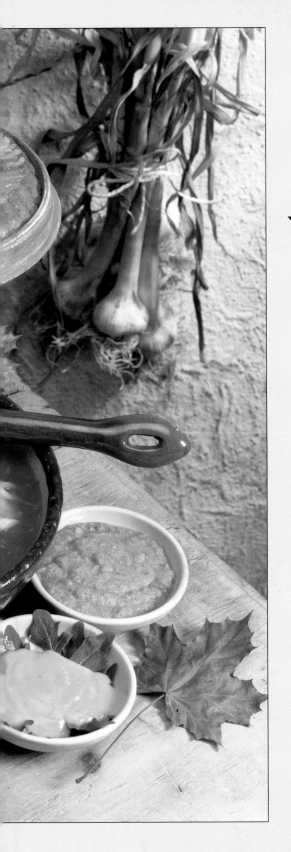

Eat
Yourself
Slim

Rosemary Conley

Century Publishing

Published by Century in 2002

5 7 9 10 8 6 4

Copyright © Rosemary Conley Enterprises, 2001

Rosemary Conley has asserted her right under the Copyright, Designs and Patents Act, 1988 to be identified as the author of this work

First published in the United Kingdom in 2001 by Century
Random House UK Limited
20 Vauxhall Bridge Road, London SW1V 2SA

Random House Australia (Pty) Limited
20 Alfred Street, Milsons Point, Sydney,
New South Wales 2061, Australia

Random House New Zealand Limited
18 Poland Road, Glenfield
Auckland 10, New Zealand

Random House (Pty) Limited
Endulini, 5a Jubilee Road, Parktown 2193, South Africa

The Random House Group Limited Reg. No. 954009
www.randomhouse.co.uk

A CIP catalogue record for this book is available
from the British Library

Papers used by Random House UK Limited are natural, recyclable products made from wood grown in sustainable forests. The manufacturing processes conform to the environmental regulations of the country of origin

ISBN 0 7126 1553 9

Photography by Peter Barry
Food styling by Dean Simpole-Clarke
Designed by Roger Walker

Printed and bound in Germany by Appl, Wemding

Also by Rosemary Conley

Rosemary Conley's Hip and Thigh Diet
Rosemary Conley's Complete Hip and Thigh Diet
Rosemary Conley's Inch Loss Plan
Rosemary Conley's Hip and Thigh Diet Cookbook
(with Patricia Bourne)
Rosemary Conley's Metabolism Booster Diet
Rosemary Conley's Whole Body Programme
Rosemary Conley's New Hip and Thigh Diet Cookbook
(with Patricia Bourne)
Shape Up for Summer
Rosemary Conley's Beach Body Plan
Rosemary Conley's Flat Stomach Plan
Be Slim! Be Fit!
Rosemary Conley's Complete Flat Stomach Plan
Rosemary Conley's New Body Plan
Rosemary Conley's New Inch Loss Plan
Rosemary Conley's Low Fat Cookbook
Rosemary Conley's Red Wine Diet
Rosemary Conley's Low Fat Cookbook Two

IMPORTANT

If you have a medical condition or are pregnant, the diet described in this book should not be followed without first consulting your doctor. All guidelines and warnings should be read carefully, and the author and publisher cannot accept responsibility for injuries or damage arising out of a failure to comply with the same.

Contents

Acknowledgements

This is my 25th book and I am only too aware that without the help of my wonderful team this latest volume would not now be in your hands.

So, a huge thank you to Dean Simpole-Clarke for creating, yet again, so many delicious, mouthwatering low-fat recipes and for recreating them so beautifully for the photographs, also to photographer Peter Barry for his expertise in illustrating the food so clearly.

Also, thank you so much to my assistant Melody Patterson who worked tirelessly for months, drawing together the various elements of the book, putting them into a readable format and for completing the nutritional analysis of every recipe and menu suggestion. My PA Louise Jones was a great help too, particularly when it came to proof reading. Thank you, Lou.

Special thanks must go to my editor, Jan Bowmer, who has, once again, provided her expertise in making this book a workable, logical volume for you, the reader, to follow. Her meticulous attention to detail never ceases to amaze me.

Thank you to Dr Susan Jebb for her invaluable help and expertise in checking that the advice and facts we give you are correct and appropriate.

To my publishers Century I say a big thank you and to art director Dennis Barker and designer Roger Walker. Also to Andy McKillop who encouraged me to write the book, and to Ron Beard for selling it so enthusiastically, through his sales team, to the retailers.

Last, but by no means least, I want to say thank you to the members of Rosemary Conley Diet and Fitness Clubs for completing the questionnaires on the effectiveness of this diet and to Ally Evans, who worked so hard in collating these results into a useable format. You did a brilliant job, Ally. Thank you.

Foreword

For many years Rosemary Conley has endeavoured to help people put their good intentions into practice with low-fat eating plans, combined with exercise, to maximise weight loss and promote good health. This approach worked because in the past most low-fat foods contained fewer calories than their high-fat equivalents. However, advances in food processing and food technology mean that today some low-fat foods contain just as many calories as the high-fat varieties. To lose weight successfully you need to cut fat *and* calories.

This book combines an individualised, calorie-controlled eating plan, together with a wealth of new low-fat recipes to make it easier and more interesting to plan your meals. Using these ideas, you can cook healthy food for the whole family, while choosing the right portions to help you cut calories and lose weight.

Dr Susan Jebb
Deputy Chair of the Association for the Study of Obesity

Useful Information

Weight conversions

All weights are given in imperial and metric. All conversions are approximate. Use only one set of measures and do not mix the two. The table below shows the conversions used.

Ounce (oz)	Pound (lb)	Gram (g)
1		25
2		50
3		75
4	$\frac{1}{4}$	115
5		150
6		175
7		200
8	$\frac{1}{2}$	225
16	1	450
	$1\frac{1}{2}$	675
	2	900

Liquid measures

1 tablespoon	= 3 teaspoons	= $\frac{1}{2}$fl oz	= 15ml
2 tablespoons	= 6 teaspoons	= 1fl oz	= 30ml
4 tablespoons	= $\frac{1}{4}$ cup	= 2fl oz	= 50ml
5 tablespoons	= $\frac{1}{3}$ cup	= $2\frac{1}{2}$fl oz	= 75ml
8 tablespoons	= $\frac{1}{2}$ cup	= 4fl oz	= 120ml
10 tablespoons	= $\frac{2}{3}$ cup	= 5fl oz	= 150ml ($\frac{1}{4}$ pint)
12 tablespoons	= $\frac{3}{4}$ cup	= 6fl oz	= 175ml
16 tablespoons	= 1 cup	= 8fl oz	= 250ml ($\frac{1}{2}$ US pint)

Note: A UK pint contains 20fl oz

American cup measures can be convenient to use, especially when making large quantities. However, although the volume remains the same, the weight may vary, as illustrated opposite.

Imperial	American
Flour	*Flour*
plain and self-raising	all purpose
1oz	1/4 cup
4oz	1 cup
Cornflour	*Cornstarch*
1oz	1/4 cup
generous 2oz	1/2 cup
4 1/2 oz	1 cup
Sugar (granulated/caster)	*Sugar (granulated)*
4oz	1/2 cup
7 1/2 oz	1 cup
Sugar (icing)	*Sugar (confectioner's)*
1oz	1/4 cup
4 1/2 oz	1 cup
Sugar (soft brown)	*Sugar (light and dark brown)*
4oz	1/2 cup firmly packed
8oz	1 cup firmly packed

Useful measures

1 egg	56ml	2fl oz
1 egg white	28ml	1fl oz
2 rounded tablespoons breadcrumbs	30g	1oz
2 level teaspoons gelatine	8g	1/4oz

1oz (25g) granular aspic sets 600ml (1 pint).
1/2oz (15g) powdered gelatine or 4 leaves sets 600ml (1 pint).

All spoon measures are level unless otherwise stated.

Wine quantities

Average serving	ml	fl oz
1 glass wine	90ml	3fl oz
1 glass port or sherry	60ml	2fl oz
1 glass liqueur	30ml	1fl oz

Oven temperature conversions

Celsius (Centigrade)	Fahrenheit	Gas Mark	Definition
130	250	$\frac{1}{2}$	very cool
140	275	1	cool
150	300	2	warm
170	325	3	moderate
180	350	4	moderate
190	375	5	moderately hot
200	400	6	hot
220	425	7	hot
230	450	8	very hot
240	475	9	very hot

Abbreviations

oz	ounce
lb	pound
kg	kilogram
fl oz	fluid ounce
ml	millilitre
C	Celsius (Centigrade)
F	Fahrenheit
kcal	kilocalorie (calorie)

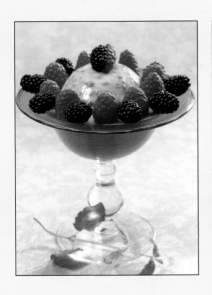

Equipment and terms

British	American
baking tin	baking pan
base	bottom
cocktail stick	toothpick
dough or mixture	batter
frying pan	skillet
greaseproof paper	waxed paper
grill/grilled	broil/broiled
knock back dough	punch back dough
liquidiser	blender
muslin	cheesecloth
pudding basin	ovenproof bowl
stoned	pitted
top and tail (gooseberries)	clean (gooseberries)
whip/whisk	beat/whip

Ingredients

British	American
aubergine	egg plant
bacon rashers	bacon slices
bicarbonate of soda	baking soda
black cherries	bing cherries
boiling chicken	stewing chicken
broad beans	fava or lima beans
capsicum pepper	sweet pepper
cauliflower florets	cauliflowerets
celery stick	celery stalk
stock cube	bouillon cube
chicory	belgium endive
chilli	chile pepper

British	American
cooking apple	baking apple
coriander	cilantro
cornflour	cornstarch
courgette	zucchini
crystallised ginger	candied ginger
curly endive	chicory
demerara sugar	light brown sugar
essence	extracts
fresh beetroot	raw beets
gelatine	gelatin
head celery	bunch celery
icing	frosting
icing sugar	confectioner's sugar
plain flour	all purpose flour
root ginger	ginger root
self-raising flour	all purpose flour sifted with baking powder
soft brown sugar	light brown sugar
spring onion	scallion
stem ginger	preserved ginger
sultanas	seedless white raisins
wholemeal	wholewheat

Introduction

This is a diet book and a low-fat cookbook, rolled into one.

I have included a tried and tested, incredibly effective diet combined with a selection of sumptuous recipes to keep your taste buds satisfied as you lose your unwanted weight, or to keep you slim if you have already achieved your goal.

The principle of the diet is somewhat different from any of my other diets as it includes an optional, daily high-fat treat which can be saved up for a bigger treat if you want to. Also the diet is based on your own personal daily calorie allowance which you will be able to calculate for yourself.

Over the last 20 months, the principle of the Eat Yourself Slim diet has been followed by members of Rosemary Conley Diet and Fitness Clubs across the UK. Around 300,000 women (and some men) have followed it and undeniably proved its effectiveness.

After they had followed the diet for six months, I asked 600 members, selected at random, to complete a questionnaire. I wanted to know the diet's effectiveness since I was now including an optional high-fat treat each day.

All my previous diet plans had strictly excluded anything high in fat. Also how did everyone feel about being a calorie counter again after shying away from them for years?

What about inch loss – was this diet as effective in that area? How did the dieters get on with their personal calorie allowance? Did they find it easy to follow?

I needn't have worried. The results were fantastic! Out of those questioned, 98 per cent said the diet was easy to follow, 78 per cent said it was the most effective diet they had ever followed and 76 per cent said they had lost more inches than ever before!

The weekly weight losses for all 600 members questioned were added together and divided by 600 to arrive at an average weekly weight loss figure. Many dieters had been on the diet for many months, some for a somewhat shorter period of time. Nevertheless, the average loss across all 600 worked out at 1.7lb per week. This is incredible when you realise that some people have only a small amount to lose and that it was taken over a wide time scale.

When asked if they lost weight faster on this diet, 67 per cent said they did, 27 per cent said that the progress was about the same with only 6 per cent saying 'no'.

When asked if they were happy with their inch loss, 1 per cent said they were disappointed, 1 per cent said they were not very happy, 17 per cent were happy, 31 per cent were very happy and 50 per cent were delighted.

Seventy-seven per cent said they were happy to count calories and 94 per cent were pleasantly surprised at how many calories they were allowed.

This book, which accompanies my TV series by the same name, offers you an extended version of the original diet plan used by our Rosemary Conley Diet and Fitness Club members. You will also find plenty of motivational tips to keep you going until you reach your weight-loss goal – and keep it off in the long term.

I have tried to give you the ultimate guide to help you achieve a trim and healthy body. If you combine the diet with some extra physical activity, you'll maximise your weight-loss progress. So enjoy the journey and revel in your ultimate success.

To encourage you, here are some comments from just a few of the trial dieters:

'This plan is definitely the one for me, as it's normal good food that's easy to buy, cook, prepare, etc. and very tasty to eat!'
Kimberley Fay, Milton Keynes

'This diet is my favourite. So uncomplicated, so much choice and good to eat. Easy to adapt for my husband. Not so much a diet but a new way of life.'
Janet West, Huddersfield

'I have never felt this good in a long time and the weight loss has given me tremendous confidence.'
Allison Baines, Co. Durham

'I can't begin to describe the changes I feel about myself – apart from the excellent weight loss I feel so much more positive. I don't feel like I'm dieting – more like at last I'm in control of my size and health.'

H.C., Surrey

'I have tried other diets, but this is the best one I have ever done. I can't believe the number of inches I have lost with the weight.'

Susan Fox , Hampshire

'I like the idea of the diet being based on your basal metabolic rate because it makes it more personal as everybody is different. My calorie allowance is very sufficient and I feel I am getting plenty to eat and do not get the urge to "snack" between meals.'

Angela Howard, Oxfordshire

'I'm losing more weight than expected. I have to pinch myself to believe it!'

Michelle Cardy, Cornwall

'I have been much more successful on this diet. I feel great and have experienced a total change in my attitude to food and exercise, which has improved my work and social life enormously!'

L.H., Dundee

'What I like about it is the fact that the calorie allowance is connected to how much you weigh. In my case, because I weighed a lot, I was pleasantly surprised by how much I was allowed initially. Also, whenever I get a new allowance I feel proud because it means that I am right on my way, so cutting down on calories doesn't seem to be such a big scare any more.'

Julie Knoblich, Essex

'I have found this diet so easy. I have never been very successful before, but this time the weight just fell off and I'm managing to keep it fairly constant.'

Laura Knight, East Sussex

Why 'Eat Yourself Slim'?

Thirty years ago I started my first slimming club, having realised that the only way to lose weight successfully was to eat more than most diets recommended. In those days doctors handed out 1,000-calorie diet sheets, which were impossible to stick to. There just wasn't enough food to eat. I conquered my own overweight problem by giving myself more calories – and sticking to it.

In 1986 I had to follow a low-fat diet because of a gallstone problem. Without realising it, my body changed shape, shedding fat from areas I had tried to slim down since puberty – namely my hips and thighs. I always have been the ultimate pear shape.

Millions of women and some men have become slimmer and healthier since they too changed to low-fat eating.

Despite many other diets being published and promoted from various corners of the world, there is no shadow of a doubt that if you want to lose weight fast and yet healthily, if you want to be lean and energetic, there is no better way than to eat a calorie-controlled, low-fat diet and combine it with increased physical activity.

Becoming more active need only mean walking for 30 minutes, three times a week – not having to run a marathon! I am always delighted though to hear how those who hate the thought of exercise at the beginning become great fans of it later.

Often we 'hate' exercise because we 'fear' it. We think: 'I'm not going to be able to go to a class – I'm not coordinated and I might pass out'. 'Imagine the embarrassment!' 'I couldn't possibly go for a jog – everyone would laugh at me!' or 'If you think I'm going to show off my fat in public, think again!'

But you are not alone. We all felt like that – I know I did. Once we get started we find we *can* cope, but to make sure that we can, the exercise has to be at *our* level. Personally I hate running, but I love walking. I hate swimming, but I love working out to music in an aerobics class – but at a *moderate level*. I have no inclination to workout at a mega level – it would be too exhausting – so I don't do it. Find *your* level and progress at your *own* pace, then hopefully you will keep doing it.

While I was asking some of the members of our classes for their responses to the new diet plan, I decided to ask them about their attitude towards exercise. Had it changed since they joined our classes? These were the results:

Of the 600 women questioned 25 per cent admitted to not enjoying exercise before attending a Rosemary Conley Diet and Fitness class. When asked how they felt now, having attended classes for some time, only 4 per cent still didn't enjoy it. So why the big turn around? They realised they could do the exercise (our classes cater for all capabilities and all of our instructors are specially trained to modify exercises when necessary), they enjoyed the friendships of fellow members just like them and, as the weeks went by, they became fitter and could do more when *they* felt they could. As their fear diminished their confidence grew and this will happen to you too.

If you don't exercise already you need to start. It doesn't have to be awful. You can exercise in so many different ways – sporting activities, just walking or gardening (mowing the lawn is great exercise), working out at an exercise class (see inside back cover for details of where our classes are held), working out to a fitness video (click on to our website for details of several of mine), join a gym, play physical games with the children, swim – there are so many things you can do. Some cost money, but lots don't.

So what is the optimum way of losing weight?

The secret of successful, long-term, weight loss is to try to make your body believe it isn't dieting. You can achieve this by eating sufficient calories to meet your bodily needs yet few enough to affect a weight loss. It means you shouldn't starve yourself or miss out on delicious food, because if you are happy with what you are eating, you are less likely to cheat, and that is what this book is all about.

First you will be able to calculate your individual calorie allowance from the tables on pages 19–20, which are based on your sex, age and weight. Next you can choose from the many low-fat, calorie-counted menu suggestions listed, including some fabulous recipes from expert chef Dean Simpole-Clarke, with whom I have worked on TV for several years. Dean totally understands my low-fat philosophy.

Plus, for the first time in one of my diet books, you are allowed a 150-calorie daily treat which is exempt from my 4% fat rule. And for anyone not familiar with the 4% fat rule, all of my diets are based on the consumption of foods that contain 4% or less fat with the exception of oily fish, which is included, as it is vital for good health.

So why, after all these years of promoting low fat have I relented and allowed a 150-calorie high-fat treat? Well, just as 30 years ago I realised that dieters lost more weight by having a higher calorie allowance because they could stick to it, two years ago I realised that many of my low-fat dieters just couldn't find the willpower to never ever eat chocolate, Häagen-Dazs or Pringles without feeling so guilty that they broke the diet completely. So, a compromise was created and, having since then tried out this theory in our Clubs, I have proved beyond a shadow of a doubt that allowing a daily treat (which can be saved up if you wish) does not adversely affect weight and fat loss but greatly increases the level of adherence to the diet.

Never have we experienced such weight-loss successes at our Clubs as we have since the introduction of this new diet (which in the classes we called the New You Plan). The key to your success is keeping to your personal calorie allowance, making sure that the calories you eat are low fat except for your treat, and that you try to increase your activity levels within your everyday lifestyle. You can still have a glass of wine or other alcoholic drink, and, depending on how many calories you have to spend, these may be taken within or outside of your treat allowance. For example, if your daily allowance is 1700 kcal, you could have 1 unit of alcohol (e.g. 1 glass of wine) in addition to your 150 kcal treat because you have sufficient calories left to enable you to eat plenty of nutritious foods to keep your body healthy. If, on the other hand, you had a daily allowance of only 1300, then to get sufficient nutrients into the body you would have to take your unit of alcohol as part of your 150-kcal treat allowance.

As you lose each stone recalculate your calorie allowance to ensure maximum progress. As your body gets smaller it needs less fuel to feed it, so your calorie requirement reduces.

How to work out your optimum calorie allowance

Basal Metabolic Rate (BMR) Table

Women aged 18–29			Women aged 30–59			Women aged 60–74		
Body Weight			*Body Weight*			*Body Weight*		
Stones	*Kilos*	*BMR*	*Stones*	*Kilos*	*BMR*	*Stones*	*Kilos*	*BMR*
7	45	1147	7	45	1208	7	45	1048
7.5	48	1194	7.5	48	1233	7.5	48	1073
8	51	1241	8	51	1259	8	51	1099
8.5	54	1288	8.5	54	1285	8.5	54	1125
9	57	1335	9	57	1311	9	57	1151
9.5	60.5	1382	9.5	60.5	1337	9.5	60.5	1176
10	64	1430	10	64	1373	10	64	1202
10.5	67	1477	10.5	67	1389	10.5	67	1228
11	70	1524	11	70	1414	11	70	1254
11.5	73	1571	11.5	73	1440	11.5	73	1279
12	76	1618	12	76	1466	12	76	1305
12.5	80	1665	12.5	80	1492	12.5	80	1331
13	83	1712	13	83	1518	13	83	1357
13.5	86	1760	13.5	86	1544	13.5	86	1382
14	89	1807	14	89	1570	14	89	1408
14.5	92	1854	14.5	92	1595	14.5	92	1434
15	95.5	1901	15	95.5	1621	15	95.5	1460
15.5	99	1948	15.5	99	1647	15.5	99	1485
16	102	1995	16	102	1673	16	102	1511
16.5	105	2043	16.5	105	1699	16.5	105	1537
17	108	2090	17	108	1725	17	108	1563
17.5	111	2137	17.5	111	1751	17.5	111	1588
18	115	2184	18	115	1776	18	115	1614
18.5	118	2231	18.5	118	1802	18.5	118	1640
19	121	2278	19	121	1828	19	121	1666
19.5	124	2325	19.5	124	1854	19.5	124	1691
20	127	2373	20	127	1880	20	127	1717

Basal Metabolic Rate (BMR) Table

Men aged 18–29			Men aged 30–59			Men aged 60–74		
Body Weight			Body Weight			Body Weight		
Stones	Kilos	BMR	Stones	Kilos	BMR	Stones	Kilos	BMR
7	45	1363	7	45	1384	7	45	1232
7.5	48	1411	7.5	48	1421	7.5	48	1270
8	51	1459	8	51	1457	8	51	1307
8.5	54	1507	8.5	54	1494	8.5	54	1345
9	57	1555	9	57	1530	9	57	1383
9.5	60.5	1602	9.5	60.5	1567	9.5	60.5	1421
10	64	1650	10	64	1603	10	64	1459
10.5	67	1698	10.5	67	1640	10.5	67	1497
11	70	1746	11	70	1676	11	70	1535
11.5	73	1794	11.5	73	1713	11.5	73	1573
12	76	1842	12	76	1749	12	76	1611
12.5	80	1890	12.5	80	1786	12.5	80	1649
13	83	1938	13	83	1822	13	83	1687
13.5	86	1986	13.5	86	1859	13.5	86	1725
14	89	2034	14	89	1895	14	89	1763
14.5	92	2082	14.5	92	1932	14.5	92	1801
15	95.5	2129	15	95.5	1968	15	95.5	1839
15.5	99	2177	15.5	99	2005	15.5	99	1877
16	102	2225	16	102	2041	16	102	1915
16.5	105	2273	16.5	105	2078	16.5	105	1953
17	108	2321	17	108	2114	17	108	1991
17.5	111	2369	17.5	111	2151	17.5	111	2028
18	115	2417	18	115	2187	18	115	2066
18.5	118	2465	18.5	118	2224	18.5	118	2104
19	121	2513	19	121	2260	19	121	2142
19.5	124	2561	19.5	124	2297	19.5	124	2180
20	127	2609	20	127	2333	20	127	2218

The secret of long-term success

There's no better feeling when you're trying to lose weight than a waistband that's now loose (such a relief from when your stomach hung over it), trousers that have fresh air between your leg and the fabric (so much more comfortable than that feeling of material being superglued to your legs), and your top showing an attractive and feminine bustline rather than a bosom that resembles an oversized pillow being squeezed into a too small pillowcase!

Following this calorie-controlled, low-fat diet will definitely enable you to lose weight. Taking regular exercise is guaranteed to help to tone up your body and speed up your weight loss. However, even a diet combined with exercise is still not enough to achieve long-term success. You need to change your *mindset* towards food and activity in general.

This change in attitude needs you to create some positive, and remove some negative, habits *as well as* following the diet and taking regular exercise.

Place a tick alongside the statements opposite if they apply to you.

None of these actions constitutes a major sin on its own; they're just 'little extras' compared with going to the sweet counter and buying a Mars bar and a Snickers and eating them both.

☐ 'I always eat everything on my plate'. (*I was made to do that as a child.*)

☐ 'With their permission, I eat other family members' leftovers at the table'. (*Shame to waste it.*)

☐ 'I sometimes eat leftovers while walking to the kitchen'. (*If no one sees me it doesn't count!*)

☐ 'I eat leftovers while alone in the kitchen'. (*Think of the starving millions.*)

☐ 'I lick the spoon from the trifle/dessert before washing it up'. (*Saves messing up the washing up water.*)

☐ 'I like to level off the remaining trifle/dessert before placing in the fridge'. (*To make it look tidier.*)

☐ 'I keep levelling off remaining trifle/dessert over next day or so'. (*To check that it hasn't 'gone off'.*)

☐ 'I occasionally slice off a sliver of cheese from the fridge when I'm feeling peckish'. (*Sometimes more than a sliver.*)

☐ 'I eat occasional sweets or chocolates when offered by a friend'. (*I don't want to appear holier-than-thou.*)

☐ 'I eat ingredients during preparation of a recipe and lick the spoon afterwards'. (*To check that it tastes OK.*)

But I bet you put a tick in more than one box. If you ticked more than seven you might as well have had the Mars bar! By these seemingly harmless actions you are effectively sabotaging your chances of success on your weight-loss campaign. One by one, try and break all these negative habits.

So now to some positive actions and activities which take little effort but have a big effect:

- Stop leaving things at the bottom of the stairs – take them up every time.
- When the TV commercials come on, get up and do something (not get food though). Go upstairs for something, wash up, dry up, put washing in, walk dog for 2 minutes, walk around garden.
- When shopping, always use the stairs not the lift or elevator. If you must use the elevator, walk up it.
- Park further away from the door when going shopping or at the gym/pool/class.
- Make a list of your exercise programme for each week. Pin it on a noticeboard and tick off each activity as you do it. Don't beat yourself up if you don't do it all. Any is better than none.
- Go walking in your lunch break – even browsing round the shops is activity.
- Stand up when making phone calls, rather than sitting down.
- Look at housework as a workout not a chore. Vacuuming, sweeping, cleaning windows are great fat burners.

- Play active games with your children (or borrow someone else's) and have fun while you burn those calories.
- Washing and polishing your car, mowing the lawn or cutting the hedge are great forms of calorie-burning exercise. Include them in your workout schedule.

So, if you work towards stopping the habits on the first list and incorporate some of the activities in the second, you'll be amazed how positively your body will respond. Follow the diet strictly and the results will be better than ever before. You *can* lose weight . You *will* lose weight but, to do it, you need the right attitude. Remember these phrases – say them out loud. 'Every extra mouthful of food I eat means I'll lose less weight' and 'Every bit of extra activity I do – no matter now small – will speed up my weight loss'. Go on, just do it!

Are you a yo-yo dieter?

One minute you have the willpower of a saint and you know that this time you're going to really stick to the diet, exercise three times a week and see fantastic results. Then, for no particular reason, you find yourself devouring a chocolate bar – or two – as though they had just been washed up on a desert island and you hadn't eaten proper food for a month! You can't eat it fast enough, it doesn't seem to touch the sides, and before you know it, down goes bar number two!

Then horror strikes. It suddenly dawns on you what you've done. You suddenly remember you're trying to lose weight. It was almost as though you didn't decide to eat the chocolate – it just found its way into your mouth. You feel gutted. You can't believe you've just done it!

'Am I going mad, perhaps?' you ask yourself. You decide you must be. You say to yourself: 'How can this sensible, intelligent, rational woman who has a responsible job, whom people respect, behave like an irresponsible idiot?'

Well, take heart, because you, and millions of women just like you, go through exactly the same emotion time and time again. It isn't about intelligence, or irresponsibility, or uselessness. It is a pain in the backside fact of life, that when you are trying to lose weight you are vulnerable. As normal, regular human beings we are open to temptation. As soon as we make some restrictions on our food intake, that 'forbidden fruit' appeals all the more. When Eve was in the Garden of Eden she could have anything she wanted except off one particular tree. So what does she do? She chooses to eat from the forbidden tree. Why? Because she was tempted, and we are no different today.

When we go on a diet we tell ourselves that we can't eat this and that (but we enjoy those things!) and that we need to exercise (but we don't like getting hot and sweaty!), so we are telling our brain: 'I've got to do all these things I don't like – and I'll probably feel hungry too – just to get slimmer! In a weak moment we throw in the towel and 'eat from the forbidden tree' because it seems like a good idea at the time. Why? Because we've told our brain only negative messages, only the disadvantages of going on a diet and fitness programme, instead of positive ones. Positive messages are words like, 'When I lose weight I'll be wearing size 12 instead of a size 18. I'll be able to join in my child's sports day without being an embarrassment. My husband will think I look more attractive – I will have so much more energy. I will look younger and feel 10 times healthier. I'll be able to wear all those clothes in the wardrobe that I've not been able to wear for ages'.

Just because you've been a yo-yo dieter in the past, doesn't mean you have to be so for ever. I used to be one and I've cured myself by eating three substantial, low-fat meals a day. I cured myself by making the rule, that if I had a binge I wouldn't skip the next meal in an attempt to cancel it. It worked. I would eat my normal, low-fat, calorie-controlled meal and put the binge behind me. One binge doesn't matter, but three binges do! Don't beat yourself up about it. You're human. You're bound to have bad days – we all do. Don't use them as an excuse to pack it in.

So, draw a line under your dieting history now. Decide today that this is a brand new start and this time, you will do it! And you can!

Facts about food and how the Eat Yourself Slim Diet works

As a guideline, I recommend you select foods with 4% or less fat – that's up to 4 grams of fat for every 100 grams of product, though there are some exceptions such as oily fish.

The 4% fat guideline is an extremely simple and effective rule of thumb, with no need to count or add up fat grams. It has been proved that following a calorie-controlled, low-fat diet is unquestionably the safest and most effective way to lose fat from the body and therefore lose weight. It really, really works.

Let me explain how. Compared with other foods such as carbohydrates and proteins, fat in the diet is very easily stored as fat on the body.

Too much fat in the diet has been proven to be harmful to health. Too little fat can be unhealthy, too, which is why we recommend you eat between 23 and 40 grams of fat a day while you are losing your excess weight but no more than 70 grams when maintaining a healthy weight. My eating plan will help you achieve this.

Get to know the nutrition labels on the packaging of all the foods that you buy. Most nutrition panels will give the quantities per 100g of product and some will give the nutrition details per serving. On the left-hand side will be the words like Energy, Protein, Carbohydrate and so on. Energy means the number of calories that the product yields and this is the figure that you need to be mindful of as far as the serving size is concerned. You have calculated your personal calorie allowance, and every item of food that you eat needs to be included in this. The only other column on the nutrition panel that you really need to look at is under 'fat' and it doesn't matter whether it's saturated or unsaturated since, as far as gaining or losing weight is concerned, fat is fat. Under the 100g column you need to select foods with 4% or less fat and this will ensure that you are following a low-fat diet. In this diet I allow you to have a 150-calorie treat that is exempt of the 4g fat rule.

If you follow the 4% rule for the rest of your food, the fat grams will look after themselves. So just keep an eye on the daily calorie intake. It is easy to eat too many low-fat foods and consequently eat too many calories and then weight loss can be very slow or non-existent. I want you to lose your weight as fast as it's healthy to do so, so calories are crucial. The total fat grams per serving are not important and I would strongly suggest that you do not get into the habit of counting fat grams as well as calories. You just don't need to.

I have created a selection of everyday meals from which you can choose to eat what you like best. All the calories have been counted for you, so you simply need to look under the different calorie headings as to whether you want a 200-calorie breakfast or one that contains 250 calories, and so on. If you stick to the calorie allowance that you have calculated from the tables on pages 19–20, you will definitely lose weight and, if you combine your eating plan with increased physical activity, you will lose weight even faster.

Each day I recommend that you eat breakfast, lunch and dinner and also consume 450ml (¾ pint) of skimmed or semi-skimmed milk. Also, of course, in your total calorie allowance there's your special treat allowance of 150 calories to consider, which can be taken daily if you wish or saved up for a special occasion each week. However, don't carry it over to the next week.

Each day your daily intake should include five portions of fruit and/or vegetables. Fruit can be eaten with or between meals but remember to include the calories in your daily total.

This eating plan has been designed to work for anyone, whatever your personal circumstances or preference for food. Just select your favourite meals from the variety of menus listed. You can easily plan ahead if you wish. Losing weight has never been easier.

If you know you will be dining out in the evening, you can save up some calories by choosing lower-calorie options for breakfast and lunch and use up your day's treat allowance too. Alternatively, you might have saved up a previous day's treat so that you can relax and indulge yourself with a clear conscience.

I understand that losing weight isn't straightforward because it can be a struggle to maintain sufficient willpower. Some people find it almost impossible to stick unfalteringly to a weight-reducing eating plan. We all need a safety valve. We need to feel we can indulge legitimately if we have a serious craving for something, without feeling we've ruined all our hard work.

As you know, each day you are allowed 150 calories as a treat. Now, while you are free to select any high-fat treat you wish within the 150-calorie allowance, it is important to understand that if you select treats that fall *within* the 4% fat rule you are likely to lose your excess weight and inches even more quickly. Depending on your personal calorie allowance, all or part of this daily treat can be taken as a dessert after your main meal or at any other time. If you wish you could also take your treat as an alcoholic drink, providing of course that you keep within the calorie allowance. Furthermore, these treat calories can be saved up over a week and used for bigger treats. So if you desperately want to eat a cream cake or even a Mars bar you can just save up a few days' worth of treats. The same applies to alcohol. If your weekends are very sociable, save up your treat allowance and enjoy a few drinks with your friends.

You might well ask: 'But will I still lose weight if I choose treats with more than 4% fat?' Well, providing you don't exceed your daily calorie allowance and you use your treat allowance accurately, yes you definitely will. But if you relax your portion sizes, nibble extras in between meals and are rather casual about your treats, you may not. Losing weight is a matter of physics. If we eat fewer calories than our body uses for energy, it's inevitable that we will lose weight. It's rather like a bank account. Every time we spend money our bank balance reduces. If we overspend we have to draw on our savings to make up the difference. It's the same with our bodies. If we spend more energy than we take in in the form of food, we draw on our savings of fat stored around our body to make up the difference.

You may also ask: 'How is it that I have to follow the 4% fat rule for the rest of the diet but not for my treat. Surely that will cause me to gain weight fast?' Providing you stick to the calorie allowance for your daily treat you can't do much damage when you balance it out against the low-fat food you are eating throughout the rest of the day. If you save up your treats for a special occasion, it means you will have gone without them on other days so it all balances out. I must stress, though, that it is better to spread them out if you can.

Basic nutrition

We need to eat a variety of foods to obtain the nutrients we need for good health. I find it easier to think of nutrients as falling into two categories – tangible and intangible. Tangible nutrients are carbohydrates, proteins and fats. Minerals and vitamins fall into the intangible category because they are found *within* carbohydrates, proteins and fats. The key to good nutrition is getting the balance right. Eating too much of one thing can be as bad as eating too little of another. Here are some basic nutritional guidelines.

Carbohydrates

Carbohydrates include foods such as bread, potatoes, rice, cereals, pasta, as well as fruit and vegetables. These foods provide bulk in the diet and will only be stored as fat on the body if eaten in great excess. One gram of carbohydrate yields 4 calories. Carbohydrate should feature as the largest component in every meal, as out of all the food groups, it is the most important supplier of energy, and 60% of the calories we consume each day should come from this food group.

Proteins

Proteins include foods such as meat, fish and poultry, eggs, cheese and milk. Their primary use is to help the body grow and to renew and repair existing tissue. It should be eaten in moderation, forming about 15% of our daily calorie intake. Too much protein can be harmful because it has to be metabolised by the kidneys, so high-protein diets are neither healthy nor recommended. If we eat more protein than we need, the excess cannot be stored by the body. Instead, part of the protein will be excreted from the body and the remainder will be used to provide energy, therefore delaying the burning of fat.

Fats

Fats include foods such as oil, butter, margarine, cream and lard. Fat is also found in varying amounts in other foods, such as cakes, biscuits, pastry and confectionery. It is a concentrated form of energy that is efficiently stored by the body for emergencies and also supplies some valuable nutrients for health. Fat contains 9 calories per gram, which is more than twice the number of calories contained in one gram of carbohydrate or protein.

On a weight-reducing diet women should allow between 23 and 40 grams per day, while men should allow between 38 and 50 grams. When seeking to maintain weight, rather than trying to lose it, the maximum fat intake should not exceed 70 grams per day for women and 100 grams per day for men.

A small amount of fat is necessary for good health, and oily fish such as salmon, mackerel and herrings contain essential fatty acids that are particularly beneficial. I recommend that you eat one portion of oily fish each week.

Minerals

There are many minerals, all of which play an important role in helping us achieve good health. In most cases, a varied and healthy diet will ensure we are not missing out. However, there are two important minerals – calcium and iron – which require special mention. Since dairy products are the richest source of calcium, and red meat is the richest source of iron, on a low-fat diet it is particularly important to make sure you are taking in sufficient amounts. If you consume 450ml (¾ pint) of skimmed or semi-skimmed milk plus a small pot of yogurt (150g/5oz) each day and eat red meat four times a week, you will probably meet your needs.

We need calcium to help maintain our bones and teeth and we need iron to make haemoglobin, which carries oxygen around the body in the red blood cells. Too little iron, and we become anaemic. Too little calcium, and we reduce the strength of our bones and risk osteoporosis. The tables on pages 30 and 31 will help you check if you are getting enough of each nutrient. If you're not, you need to amend your diet accordingly.

Please note, these tables are intended as a rough guide only, since the iron and calcium content of foods may differ slightly with different cuts of meat and different brands of cereals, especially if they have been fortified.

Vitamins

Vitamins fall into two categories: fat-soluble and water-soluble. Vitamins A, D, E and K are fat-soluble and do not need to be consumed daily, since the body is able to store them. However, the B complex vitamins and vitamin C are water-soluble. Since these cannot be stored by the body, they need to be consumed daily. Each vitamin has its own special function and all are essential for good health.

Even though my diets are designed to be healthy and balanced, I do recommend you take a multivitamin tablet daily, just to make doubly sure you have all the vitamins you need. This will ensure that you always get all the micronutrients your body needs.

These days much attention has been focused on the antioxidant vitamins (vitamins A, C, and E). These vitamins help to zap the free radicals that occur naturally in the body. For thousands of years, the balance between antioxidants and free radicals in the body has been just fine, naturally. But now, with increased pollution, radiation from microwaves, TVs and computers and even electric light bulbs, as well as increased exposure to stress, the body is producing more free radicals. These are the bad guys. To neutralise them, we need to increase the number of antioxidants (the good guys) by eating more of the foods that contain the ACE vitamins. They're easy to spot because many of these vitamins are found in brightly coloured vegetables and fruit. Other chemical compounds in fruit and vegetables, known as flavonoids, also act as antioxidants. Flavonoids are found in red wine too. Some minerals, such as zinc and selenium, can also act as antioxidants.

So, make sure you eat a wide range of foods to get all the vitamins and minerals you need. If in doubt, consider taking a micronutrient (vitamin/mineral) supplement.

Women planning to conceive should take an extra supplement of folic acid to reduce the risk of having a baby with a neural tube defect such as spina bifida.

Alcohol

Alcohol is a mixture of good and bad. It is a relaxant and has been acknowledged by the medical profession as having a real benefit in relieving stress. Alcohol in moderate quantities also helps to reduce the risk of heart disease. It is, nevertheless, a mild form of poison and the body works hard to get rid of it. On most of my diets, I allow a single unit of alcohol each day for women and two for men. Remember, too, that alcohol can be addictive, and we need to be mindful of the dangers. As with all things, moderation is the key.

There has been much debate and also many trials to determine the benefits and disadvantages of consuming alcohol, ranging from whether it helps your heart to whether it makes you fat. It was even suggested at one point that the calories from alcohol didn't count because the body processes calories from alcohol in a different way from other calories. But alcohol calories do count.

In its neat form, alcohol yields 7 calories per gram, but of course we never consume alcohol in its pure state. It is always diluted by water, even in the strongest spirits. The calories in your favourite tipple may not always be directly related to the alcohol content, since many drinks contain sugar, carbohydrate and sometimes even fat.

Alcohol is easily absorbed by the stomach, but the only way the body can rid itself of alcohol is by burning it in the liver and other tissues. Since alcohol is essentially a toxin and the body has no useful purpose for storing it, the body prioritises the elimination of it at the cost of processing other foods you have eaten. Consequently, other foods may be converted to fat more readily than usual, thereby increasing your fat stores.

In the many trials I have carried out for my diets I have always found that slimmers who do drink a little alcohol while following the diet do at least as well as those who don't and, in some cases, lose more weight. But rather than suggesting that alcohol has any miracle effect, I believe it's down to the fact that if you are allowed a drink you feel less restricted, can still socialise and feel as if you are leading a 'normal' life.

Iron content of foods

Food	Serving size	mg
Liver	100g cooked weight	8
Kidney	100g cooked weight	7
Venison	100g cooked weight	8
Lean beef	100g cooked weight	3
Lean lamb	100g cooked weight	2
Pork	100g cooked weight	1
Ham	100g cooked weight	1
Duck	100g cooked weight	3
Chicken/turkey	100g cooked weight	1
Egg	1	1
Chickpeas	100g cooked weight	2
Lentils	100g cooked weight	2.5
Baked beans	1 small can	2
Potatoes	100g	0.5
Spinach	50g cooked weight	2
Watercress	50g	1
Cabbage	50g cooked weight	0.5
Broccoli	50g cooked weight	0.5
Dried fruit	50g	1
White bread	1 slice	0.5
Wholemeal bread	1 slice	0.8
Branflakes	25g	7 (fortified)
Weetabix	25g	4 (fortified)

The reference nutrient intake (RNI) for the female population is 14.8mg per day and 8.7mg for the male population.

Calcium content of foods

Food	Weight	mg
Milk	600ml	680
Cheddar cheese	25g	225
Cottage cheese	1 small pot	60
Yogurt	1 small pot	360
Egg	1	25
Sardines	50g cooked weight	250
Pilchards (canned)	50g	150
Prawns	50g cooked weight	75
Tofu	100g	500
Ice cream	50g	70
White bread	1 slice	30 (fortified)
Wholemeal bread	1 slice	7
Weetabix	25g	10
Shredded wheat	25g	12
Spinach	50g cooked weight	300
Watercress	50g	110
Dried fruit	50g	30

The reference nutrient intake (RNI) for both the female and male population is 700mg per day (800mg per day for 15- to 18-year-olds).

The key is to have a little each day, rather than drinking a lot on the occasional drinking binge. Perhaps the greatest danger from drinking alcohol when you are dieting is that it is extremely effective at diluting your willpower. Because it is a relaxant, it's so easy to think, 'Oh, what the heck, I'll diet tomorrow', and then really overindulge on the food front!

Reading nutrition labels

Nowadays we are fortunate that most food products we buy contain lots of useful information on the nutrition label. This provides us with a breakdown of their nutritional content as well as the number of calories and amount of fat. To simplify matters, as far as weight control is concerned, the two key things to look at are energy and fat.

The figure relating to 'energy' tells you the number of calories in 100g of the product (you can ignore the kJ figure – just look at the kcal one). You then need to calculate how much of the product you will actually be eating to work out the number of calories per portion.

The fat content may be broken down into polyunsaturates and saturates but, for anyone on a weight-reducing diet, this is not significant. It is the total fat content per 100g that is relevant in our calculations. I make the general

NUTRITIONAL INFORMATION	
	Per 100g
ENERGY	172 kJ/40 kcal
PROTEIN	1.8g
CARBOHYDRATE	8.0g
(of which sugars)	(2.0g)
FAT	0.2g
(of which saturates)	(Trace)
FIBRE	1.5g
SODIUM	0.3g

and simple rule that my dieters should only select foods where the label shows the fat content as 4g or less fat per 100g of product, i.e. 4% or less fat. I believe the actual amount of fat per portion is of lesser importance. If you follow the simple 4% fat rule and restrict your calorie intake to a number equivalent to your basal metabolic rate (see pages 19–20), the fat content of your food will look after itself. The only exceptions to this rule are your daily 150-calorie treat, lean cuts of meat such as beef, lamb and pork, which may be just over the 4% yardstick, and oily fish such as salmon and mackerel. In some recipes occasional high-fat ingredients have been used in very small quantities to introduce a special flavour or texture. As most recipes serve 4 people, the amount of fat is negligible.

Cooking the low-fat way

To cook the low-fat way you will need some basic non-stick kitchen essentials such as a non-stick frying pan or wok, some non-stick baking tins and the appropriate utensils to go with them. The first time you cook a stir-fry in a non-stick wok without a drop of oil is quite a revelation. The moisture that comes from the meat and vegetables prevents the food from sticking or tasting dry.

Once you have got used to low-fat cooking there will be no turning back. It really is easier than you think. In the following pages I have included advice on the kind of equipment you need and how to care for it, as well as outlining the various low-fat cooking techniques and suggestions for flavour enhancers to help your food taste delicious.

Equipment you will need

Utensils

At one time, non-stick surfaces used to have a very short lifespan before becoming scratched and worn. Fortunately, in recent years great progress been made with non-stick pans, although the old adage 'you get what you pay for' still holds firm. Buy a cheap non-stick pan, and the first time you slightly burn the pan, the surface begins to peel.

It is worth investing in a top-quality non-stick wok and a non-stick frying pan, both with lids. I use these two pans more than anything else in my kitchen. The lid is crucial, since this allows the contents of the pan to steam which adds moisture to the dish.

Non-stick saucepans are useful, too, for cooking sauces, porridge, scrambled eggs and other foods that tend to stick easily. Lids are essential for these too. Also, treat yourself to a set of non-stick baking tins and trays. Cakes, Yorkshire puddings, scones, and lots more can all be cooked the low-fat way.

To clean a non-stick pan, always soak the pan first to loosen any food that is still inside, then wash with a non-abrasive sponge or cloth. Any brush or gentle scourer used carefully will do the trick of cleaning away every particle without effort and without damage to the surface. Allowing pans to boil dry is the biggest danger for non-stick pans, so, when cooking vegetables, keep an eye on the water levels!

Non-scratch implements

Wooden spoons and spatulas, Teflon (or similar) coated tools and others marked as suitable for use with non-stick surfaces are a must. If you continue to use metal forks, spoons and spatulas, you will scratch and spoil the non-stick surface of pans. Treat the surfaces kindly, and good non-stick pans will last for years.

Other equipment

You will no doubt already have some of the items listed below, but I have made the list as comprehensive as possible, including the things I use most often.

Aluminium foil
Baking parchment
Chopping boards (1 small, 1 medium, 1 large)
Clingfilm
Colander (1 small and 1 large)
Fish kettle (stainless steel)
Flour shaker
Food processor
Garlic press
Good quality can opener
Juicer
Kitchen paper
Kitchen scales (ones that weigh small amounts accurately)
Lemon squeezer
Measuring jugs ($1 \times \frac{1}{2}$ litre/1 pint, 1×1 litre/ 2 pints)
Melon baller
Mixing bowls (1×1 litre/2 pints, 1×2 litres/ 4 pints, 1×4 litres/8 pints)
Multi-surface grater
Ovenproof dishes
Palette knife

Pasta spoon (non-scratch)

Pastry brush

Pepper mill

Pizza cutter

Plastic containers with lids

Potato masher (non-scratch)

Ramekin dishes

Rolling pin

Scissors

Set of sharp knives (all sizes)

Sieve (1 small and 1 large)

Slotted spoon (non-scratch)

Steamer

Vegetable peeler

Whisk (balloon type)

Wire rack

Zester

Store cupboard

There are many items that are very useful to have in stock. Build up your store cupboard over a period of time to avoid a marathon shopping trip!

Arrowroot

Cornflour

Plain flour

Self-raising flour

Gelatine

Marmite

Bovril

Dried herbs

Tomato ketchup

HP sauce

Fruity sauce

Barbecue sauce

Reduced oil salad dressing

Balsamic vinegar

White wine vinegar

Black peppercorns

Salt

White pepper

Vegetable stock cubes

Chicken stock cubes

Beef stock cubes

Lamb stock cubes

Pork stock cubes

Long-grain easy cook rice

Basmati rice

Pasta

Oats

Tabasco sauce

Soy sauce

Worcestershire sauce

Caster sugar

Brown sugar

Artificial sweetener

fresh items

Eggs

Fresh herbs

Garlic

Lemons

Oranges

Tomatoes

Low-fat cooking techniques

Dry-frying meat and poultry

The secret of dry-frying is to have your non-stick pan over the correct heat. If it's too hot, the pan will dry out the food too soon and the contents will burn. If the heat is too low, you lose the crispness recommended for a stir-fry. Practice makes perfect and a simple rule is to preheat the pan until it is quite hot (but not too hot!) before adding any of the ingredients. Test if the pan is hot enough by adding a piece of meat or poultry. The pan is at the right temperature if the meat sizzles on contact. Add the rest of the meat or poultry and toss it around. Once it is sealed on all sides (when it changes colour) you can reduce the heat a little as you add your seasonings, followed by vegetables and any other ingredients.

Cooking meat and poultry is simple, as the natural fat and juices run out almost immediately, providing plenty of moisture to prevent burning.

When cooking mince, I dry-fry it first and place it in a colander to drain away any fat that has emerged. I wipe out the pan with kitchen paper to remove any fatty residue and then return the meat to the pan to continue cooking my shepherd's pie or bolognese sauce.

Dry-frying vegetables

Vegetables contain their own juices and soon release them when they become hot, so dry-frying works just as well for vegetables as it does for meat and poultry. When dry-frying vegetables, it's important not to overcook them. They should be crisp and colourful so that they retain their flavour and most of their nutrients. Perhaps the most impressive results are with onions. When they are dry-fried, after a few minutes they go from being raw to translucent and soft and then on to become brown and caramelised. They taste superb and look for all the world like fried onions but taste so much better without all that fat.

Good results are also obtained when dry-frying large quantities of mushrooms, as they 'sweat' and make lots of liquid. Using just a few mushrooms produces a less satisfactory result unless you are stir-frying them with lots of other vegetables. If you are using a small quantity, therefore, you may find it preferable to cook them in vegetable stock.

Alternatives to frying with fat

Wine, water, soy sauce, wine vinegar, balsamic vinegar, and even fresh lemon juice all provide liquid in which food can be cooked. Some thicker types of sauces can dry out too fast if added early on in cooking, but these can be added later when there is more moisture in the pan.

When using wine or water, make sure the pan is hot before adding the other ingredients so that they sizzle in the hot pan.

Flavour enhancers

Low-fat cooking can be bland and dry, so it's important to add moisture and/or extra flavour to compensate for the lack of fat.

I have found that adding freshly ground black pepper to just about any savoury dish is a real flavour enhancer. You need a good pepper mill and you should buy your peppercorns whole and in large quantities. Ready ground black pepper is nowhere near as good. Sometimes it has other things mixed with the ground pepper, so give this one a miss.

When cooking rice, pasta and vegetables, I always add a vegetable stock cube to the cooking water. Although the stock cube does contain a little fat, the amount that is absorbed by the food is negligible and the benefit in flavour is very noticeable. I always save the water I've used to cook vegetables to make soups, gravy and sauces. Again, the fat from the stock cube that will be contained in a single serving is very small.

When making sandwiches, spread sauces such as Branston, mustard, horseradish and low-fat or fat-free dressings straight onto the bread. This helps the inside of the sandwich to stay 'put' and, because these sauces or dressings are quite highly flavoured, you won't miss the butter. Make sure you use fresh bread for maximum taste.

Here is a quick reference list of ingredients or cooking methods that can be substituted for traditional high-fat ones.

Cheese sauces Use small amounts of low-fat Cheddar, a little made-up mustard and skimmed milk with cornflour.

Custard Use custard powder and follow the instructions on the packet, using skimmed milk and artificial sweetener in place of sugar to save calories.

Cream Instead of double cream or whipping cream, use 0% fat Greek yogurt or low-fat fromage frais. Do not boil. For single cream, substitute low-fat natural or vanilla-flavoured yogurt or fromage frais.

Cream cheese Use Quark (skimmed soft cheese).

Creamed potatoes Mash the potatoes in the normal way and add fromage frais in place of butter or cream. Season well.

French dressing Use two parts apple juice to one part wine vinegar, and add a teaspoon of Dijon mustard.

Mayonnaise Use fromage frais mixed with two parts cider vinegar to one part lemon juice, plus a little turmeric and sugar.

Marie Rose dressing Use reduced oil salad dressing mixed with yogurt, tomato ketchup and a dash of Tabasco sauce and black pepper.

Porridge Cook with water and make to a sloppy consistency. Cover and leave overnight. Reheat before serving and serve with cold milk and sugar or honey.

Roux Make a low-fat roux by adding dry plain flour to a pan containing the other ingredients and 'cooking off' the flour. Then add liquid to thicken. Alternatively, use cornflour mixed with cold water or milk. Bring to the boil and cook for 2–3 minutes.

Thickening for sweet sauces Arrowroot, slaked in cold water or juice, is good because it becomes translucent when cooked.

Herbs

Herbs are fine fragrant plants that have been used to enhance and flavour food since the development of the art of cookery. As well as adding the finishing touches to a dish, many are attributed with hidden medicinal strengths that contribute to our wellbeing. Never before has there been such a wide variety of herbs introduced to our palate, from Mediterranean influences and worldwide cultures. You can buy them fresh, freeze-dried or dried, or grow your own. They all have an important role to play. Since dried herbs have a stronger flavour, they should be used more sparingly than fresh ones.

Fresh herbs fall into two categories: hard wood and soft leaf. Generally, hard wood herbs, such as rosemary, thyme and bay, are added at the beginning of a recipe in order to allow the herbs to soften and release their flavours. Soft leaf herbs, such as parsley, chervil, and basil, have more delicate flavours and are added near the end of cooking time so that they retain their flavour.

Spices

Spices were originally used to disguise ill-flavoured meat and sour foods as a result of insufficient means of chilled storage. Mainly derived from distant shores such as Sri Lanka and the East Indies, spices have over the years developed into flavour-enhancing additions. Today, they are appreciated for their aroma, colour and ability to blend together to give unique flavours.

Since spices are made from seeds, they are quite high in fat. However, because of the relatively small quantities used in recipes, their fat content is insignificant.

Spices can be kept longer than herbs, although once opened they will deteriorate. Keep out of direct sun and seal well after use.

The strongest flavours are achieved by grinding fresh seeds or whole spices as opposed to buying them already ground.

Always add spices at the beginning of a recipe, as they need to be allowed to 'cook out' to allow the flavour to develop fully. Berries such as juniper need to be crushed before cooking to release their flavours, whereas some spices such as fennel or cumin seeds benefit from being toasted in a non-stick pan.

The best way is to experiment with different spices, adding them in tiny quantities, to give a unique flavour to your cookery.

Further food tips

Rice

Rice is a nutritious, energy-giving carbohydrate food which is cheap to buy, convenient to cook and a great standby to have in your store cupboard. 25g (that's 1oz) dry weight rice gives you 100 calories. When it is cooked it will weigh 65g (2½oz). If you want to lose weight you should monitor the quantity carefully and stick to the portion sizes given. Other family members can of course eat more. Enhance the flavour of your boiled rice by adding a vegetable stock cube to the cooking water. First bring the water to the boil, then add the stock cube and then the rice. I find 'easycook' long-grain rice is the best, as it doesn't require any rinsing once it's been cooked and keeps hold of some of the flavour from the stock cube.

Pasta

Pasta is another useful high-energy carbohydrate. It is low in fat and comes in all shapes and sizes, giving great versatility to your meal planning. 25g (1oz) dry weight pasta gives you 80 calories and weighs 75g (3oz) when cooked. Watch the portion sizes while you are trying to lose weight. Family members who are not on a weight-reducing diet can of course have larger portions. As with rice and vegetables, you can enhance the flavour of pasta by adding a vegetable stock cube to the cooking water before adding the pasta. This removes the need to add butter or oil during cooking or serving.

Yogurt

Yogurt is a great low-fat protein food. It comes in so many different flavours these days and is a great aid to any menu. Although most yogurt

falls within the 4% fat rule, the calorie content can vary significantly because of its sugar content. Always check the calories per pot from the nutrition label before you buy. For a thicker, creamier natural yogurt, try 0% Greek yogurt, and if you're buying natural fromage frais, look for the Normandy variety, which is creamier, smoother and more luxurious.

Milk

On the diet you can have skimmed or semi-skimmed milk. Skimmed milk is excellent if you like it because it contains less fat and fewer calories than semi-skimmed or full-fat milk. The only problem is that many people find skimmed milk too watery – I know I do – and prefer semi-skimmed milk, which is 2% fat. This is perfectly acceptable on a weight-reducing plan. Milk is our main source of calcium and we need to drink 450ml (¾ pint) milk each day in order to obtain sufficient quantities. Both skimmed and semi skimmed milk contain more calcium than the full-fat milk. If you don't like milk you will need to take a calcium supplement. Ask your pharmacist for advice. Alternatively you could eat 3 × 150g pots of low-fat yogurt, but the total calories should not exceed 200 for all three.

Spreads, sauces and dressings

I recommend that you make your sandwiches without butter on your bread, so you may like to use some of the low-fat sauces listed earlier to moisten the bread and to help hold the filling intact. If you really can't bear your bread without low-fat spread, find one that is no more than 5% fat and use sparingly. If you must use butter or polyunsaturated margarine, deduct the calories from your 150-calorie daily treat allowance.

There are lots of sauces, such as tomato ketchup, mustard, BBQ sauce, pickle, HP fruity sauce, that are really useful to spice up your food and add moisture. Any 95% fat free salad dressing is acceptable, too, and some reduced-oil salad dressings up to 9% fat can be used in moderation. Tartare and horseradish sauce can also be taken in moderation. If any of these are used in small quantities there is no need to count the calories.

Fruit and vegetables

Fruit and vegetables are very important for good health and have an important part to play with any diet plan. You should aim to eat at least five portions of fruit and/or vegetables each day. One portion means approximately 115g (4oz). If you take your fruit in juice form, 150ml or a quarter of a pint will give you an average of 50 calories per portion. So your recommended daily intake could be taken as an apple and a pear, or perhaps 115g (4oz) grapes and 115g (4oz) strawberries, plus a salad and/or vegetables at lunch or dinner.

To enhance the flavour of vegetables during cooking, place a vegetable stock cube in the cooking water. If you do this there is no need to add salt and the cooking water is great for making gravy.

Just remember to count the calories of your fruit and vegetables into your daily total of calories. If vegetables are included in the menus listed, there is no need to count the calories, as they are already included in the meal calculations.

Drinks

It is important to drink sufficient fluids to stay healthy. I recommend that you drink as much water as possible and, of course, it's calorie free. I don't believe it matters whether it's carbonated or still. Diet drinks are also allowed freely on this weight-reducing plan. You can also drink unlimited quantities of tea and coffee, using the milk from your daily allowance. If you take sugar in your drinks you need to remember to include the calories in your daily allowance.

Alcoholic drinks are also permissible, but the calories for those should be taken from your treat allowance unless you have a higher daily allowance of calories than 1400.

It's important to be aware that, while fruit juices are healthy, they are quite high in calories. However, you could drink 150ml (1/4 pint) in place of a fruit portion, if you wish.

The Eat Yourself Slim diet

I hope you will find this diet the easiest healthy eating plan ever. Before you start you must calculate your personal calorie allowance as directed on pages 19–20. This allowance is based on the number of calories that you would burn up if you stayed in bed all day, doing absolutely nothing. Eating sufficient calories each day to meet this basic requirement will help your body believe it isn't dieting, which in turn helps to maintain your metabolic rate – that's the rate at which you burn food. If you stick closely to this calorie allowance, the great news is that every bit of physical activity that you do once you get out of bed in the morning is going to be fuelled from the fat stores around your body, so the more active you are, the more calories you will burn and the more weight you will lose.

All you have to do is select a breakfast, lunch, dinner and dessert of your choice from the already calorie counted meal suggestions so that the total doesn't exceed your daily allowance. Remember to include in your daily total the 200 calories for your milk allowance and your 150-calorie treat if you have it. If you eat fruit or anything else outside of meal times you must include the calories in your total. If you have plenty of calories to play with because of your age or weight, you can always select a meal and then supplement it with more bread, rice, pasta, fruit, or whatever. But remember, high-fat foods can only be taken from your treat allowance.

As I have explained earlier, there is no need to worry about the total fat grams per portion in a recipe, as most of the ingredients will be 4% fat or less. The exception to this is oily fish, which is higher than 4% but needs to be included for good health. There is also the occasional ingredient such as low-fat Cheddar cheese, which, even in small quantities, can make a tasty low-fat vegetarian dish.

This diet is wholly versatile. If you would like one of the lunches for your main evening meal you can have it. You can increase or reduce the serving size, you can add or subtract different accompaniments. The secret is to make it work for you and it will do if you keep within your calorie allowance.

I want to help you achieve real success so that you'll never look back. I want you to experience happiness, confidence and, most importantly, better health for you and your family in the future. If you adopt this way of eating long term, you will be making a very great step forward. On the next few pages I offer you a selection of meals which have been calorie counted for your convenience.

The diet
(V) = suitable for vegetarians

Daily allowance
450ml ($\frac{3}{4}$ pint) skimmed or semi-skimmed milk
1 × 150-calorie treat

BREAKFASTS

150-calorie breakfasts

1 (V) 2 slices light bread, toasted, plus 2 teaspoons honey, marmalade or preserve

2 (V) 50g (2oz) portion of any unsweetened bran cereal served with milk from allowance and 1 teaspoon sugar

3 (V) Fresh fruit platter, approximately 350g (12oz) in weight, of any fresh fruit of your choice in addition to your allowance

4 (V) 1 medium banana chopped into 1 low-fat yogurt (maximum 70 kcal)

5 (V) $\frac{1}{2}$ grapefruit; 1 small egg, boiled or poached, served on 1 slice light bread, toasted

6 (V) 30g (1 $\frac{1}{4}$oz) portion of any chocolate-coated cereal served with milk from allowance, plus 1 piece fresh fruit of your choice excluding bananas

7 (V) 30g (1¼oz) portion of any sugar-coated cereal served with milk from allowance; 1 piece fresh fruit

8 (V) 2 × 100g pots of low-fat yogurt (maximum 150 kcal in total)

9 (V) 1 small banana sliced, 50g (2oz) strawberries, sliced and mixed with 1 × 100g low-fat yogurt or fromage frais (maximum 70 kcal)

10 (V) 2 slices light bread, toasted, topped with 2 heaped tablespoons baked beans

250-calorie breakfasts

1 1 × 50g (2oz) bread roll spread with mustard or pickle and filled with 75g (3oz) wafer thin ham, pastrami or chicken

2 (V) 50g (2oz) porridge oats cooked with water and served with milk from allowance, 2 teaspoons honey or brown sugar

3 1 egg, dry-fried or poached, served with 2 turkey rashers plus unlimited grilled mushrooms and tomatoes and 1 medium slice wholemeal toast

4 (V) 2 M&S pikelets, toasted and spread with 1 teaspoon preserve of your choice and topped with 2 teaspoons low-fat Greek yogurt

5 (V) 50g (2oz) portion of sweetened muesli served with milk from allowance and topped with 1 chopped apple

6 2 slices light bread, toasted, topped with 1 small can (205g) baked beans plus 1 grilled turkey rasher

7 (V) 225g (8oz) fresh cherries plus 1 × 150g pot low-fat yogurt, any flavour (maximum 150 kcal)

8 (V) 2 medium slices wholemeal toast spread with 2 teaspoons marmalade or preserve

9 (V) ½ a melon seeded and filled with 115g (4oz) fresh raspberries and topped with 1 × 150g pot of low-fat yogurt of your choice (maximum 150 kcal)

10 (V) 1 medium banana, 115g (4oz) strawberries plus 1 × 150g low-fat yogurt or fromage frais, any flavour

LUNCHES
250-calorie lunches

1 3 slices light wholemeal bread spread with low-calorie reduced-fat salad dressing and filled with unlimited salad vegetables plus 25g (1oz) wafer thin ham or chicken or beef or low-fat cottage cheese

2 50g (2oz) salmon, mackerel or trout, 1 teaspoon horseradish sauce plus large salad tossed in 2 teaspoons reduced-fat salad dressing; 1 banana

3 (V) 350g (12oz) chopped salad vegetables (e.g. peppers, onions, tomatoes, cucumber, celery, carrots, baby sweetcorn) with soy

sauce to taste plus 1 chicken drumstick (all skin removed) or 1 small can (205g) baked beans

4 (V) 1 × 115g (4oz) jacket potato topped with 50g (2oz) cottage cheese mixed with 2 garlic cloves, crushed, 1/2 teaspoon dried mixed herbs and 1 teaspoon low-fat natural fromage frais or yogurt, plus large salad tossed in fat free dressing

5 (V) 2 × 48g soft brown bread rolls, filled with salad and 50g (2oz) low-fat cottage cheese

6 (V) Any prepacked sandwich or snack with no more than 250 calories and 4% fat

7 1 medium wholemeal pitta slit open and filled first with shredded lettuce then topped with 50g (2oz) tuna (in brine) mixed with 25g (1oz) canned sweetcorn and 1 teaspoon reduced-fat salad dressing

8 (V) Cream of asparagus soup (page 62) served with 50g (2oz) French bread plus 1 piece fresh fruit

9 (V) Simple tomato and roast garlic soup (page 60) served with 115g (4oz) French bread, plus 1 low-fat yogurt (maximum 70 kcal)

10 Black bean and smoked bacon soup (page 61) served with 1 slice light bread

11 (V) Sweetcorn and red pepper soup (page 66) served with 50g (2oz) French bread and 1 large banana

12 (V) Spiced cauliflower soup (page 72) served with 50g (2oz) French bread, and 1 low-fat yogurt (maximum 70 kcal)

13 (V) Sundried tomato hummus with roasted summer vegetables (page 168) plus 1 medium banana

14 (V) Potato and spinach soufflé (page 124) served with a mixed salad and 1 piece fresh fruit

15 Hattie's crunchy baked chicken (page 97) served with a large mixed salad tossed in oil free dressing, plus 1 piece fresh fruit

16 (V) 2 Roasted pepper tarts (page 158) served with a large mixed salad tossed in oil-free dressing

17 (V) Spanish omelette (page 133) served with a green side salad

18 (V) 3 pieces of any fresh fruit, 1 medium banana and 1 pot low-fat yogurt (maximum 70 kcal)

300-calorie lunches

1 Lobster couscous salad (page 108) served with chopped green salad topped with cherry tomatoes

2 Red Thai beef (page 86) served with 25g (1oz) [dry weight] boiled rice and a side salad

3 Salt cod and red pepper brandade (page 168) served with 50g (2oz) crusty bread

4 Smoked mackerel and sweet mustard pâté (page 166) served with 2 slices light bread, toasted

5 Omelette made with 2 eggs whisked together with a little milk. Season well and cook in a non-stick frying pan. When half-cooked, add unlimited peas, sweetcorn, chopped peppers and 50g (2oz) diced cooked ham. Serve with salad

6 Griddled swordfish with tomato and lime salsa (page 111) served with 115g (4oz) new potatoes, plus salad; 1 kiwi fruit

7 (V) Any prepacked readymade wholemeal sandwich with up to 300 kcal or 250 kcal plus 1 apple or pear

8 1 medium jacket potato (approximately 180g) topped with one of the following:
  - (V) 50g (2oz) baked beans, plus salad
  - (V) 50g (2oz) low-fat cottage cheese (with flavourings if desired), plus salad
  - 50g (2oz) salmon or tuna (in brine) mixed with reduced-oil salad dressing, plus salad

9 4 slices 'light' wholemeal bread spread with Waistline or similar dressing. Fill with mixed salad ingredients plus 115g (4oz) wafer thin ham, chicken, beef, turkey or 150g (5oz) low-fat cottage cheese

10 French bread margarita (page 130) served with a large salad tossed in low-fat dressing

11 Minted green pea and cucumber soup (page 168) served with 50g (2oz) crusty bread and 2 piece fresh fruit

12 Thai noodle soup (page 78) plus 1 piece fresh fruit and 1 × 150g (5oz) pot low-fat yogurt (maximum 70 kcal)

13 Celeriac and nutmeg soup (page 74) with 50g (2oz) crusty bread plus 2 pieces fresh fruit.

14 (V) Papaya, beansprout and hot banana salad (page 192), plus Lime cheesecake ice cream (page 150)

15 (V) Quick vegetable korma (page 118) served with 50g (2oz) [dry weight] boiled rice

16 (V) Honey roast corn on the cob (page 193) served with chopped salad and 25g (1oz) crusty bread

DINNERS

400-calorie dinners

1 Hot pan smoked duck with orange salad (page 106) served with 175g (6oz) new potatoes and unlimited other vegetables of your choice

2 225g (8oz) any white fish cooked without fat and served with 225g (8oz) potatoes plus unlimited other vegetables and low-fat parsley sauce

3 115g (4oz) salmon cooked without fat and served with 175g (6oz) potatoes plus unlimited other vegetables and 2 teaspoons tartare sauce

4 115g (4oz) lean lamb or pork steak (all visible fat removed) served with 115g (4oz) new potatoes plus unlimited other vegetables and low-fat gravy

5 3 low-fat sausages (max 4% fat) served with 115g (4oz) mashed potatoes plus unlimited other vegetables and low-fat gravy

6 175g (6oz) calf's or lamb's liver, braised with onions in low-fat gravy served with 115g (4oz) mashed potatoes and unlimited other vegetables of your choice

7 (V) Cherry tomato and courgette tarte tatin (page 122) served with Garlic and herb roasted new potatoes (page 195), plus a large mixed salad tossed in oil-free dressing

8 Seafood pie (page 114) served with 50g (2oz) French bread and a green salad

9 (V) Any 95% fat free readymeal (maximum 400 kcal including accompaniments)

10 (V) 1 dry-fried egg, 3 grilled turkey rashers or 1 vegetarian burger, 3 grilled tomatoes, 115g (4oz) mushrooms boiled in vegetable stock, plus 175g (6oz) 95% fat-free oven chips and 115g (4oz) peas served with sauce of your choice

11 (V) Spiced creamy vegetables with coconut milk (page 126) served with 25g (1oz) [dry weight] boiled rice, sweet mango chutney and cucumber salad

12 (V) Aubergine and spinach pasta bake (page 142) served with unlimited vegetables excluding potatoes

13 Jamaican jerk chicken (page 98) served with a small green salad

14 Pot roast lamb with celery and peppers (page 94) served with 115g (4oz) potatoes

500-calorie dinners

1 Stir-fried chicken (serves 4): chop 450g (1lb) skinned chicken breasts and season well. Dry-fry in a non-stick pan with unlimited chopped mushrooms, peppers, onion, mange tout (or any vegetables of your choice) until half-cooked. Add 1 jar of any readymade sauce (max. 4% fat) and heat thoroughly. Serve with boiled rice (50g/2oz dry weight per person)

2 1 × 175g (6oz) gammon steak grilled, served with 1 slice pineapple, pineapple sauce plus 175g (6oz) potatoes and unlimited vegetables. To make a pineapple sauce, thicken pineapple juice with cornflour or arrowroot mixed with a little cold water and cook for 2 minutes

3 Pork Provençale (page 89) served with 175g (6oz) potatoes and unlimited other vegetables

4 Preserved lemon chicken (page 100) served with 50g (2oz)[dry-weight] rice and 225g (8oz) other seasonal vegetables

5 Balsamic pork chop with tangerine (page 91) served with 175g (6oz) potatoes and 300g (10oz) other seasonal vegetables

6 Coconut roasted sea bass wrapped in banana leaves (page 180) served with unlimited vegetables excluding potatoes

7 115 (4oz) lean steak, grilled, served with 115g (4oz) jacket potato or new potatoes plus grilled tomatoes, mushrooms cooked in stock and unlimited other vegetables

8 2 lamb chops or steaks trimmed of all visible fat, grilled and served with 115g (4oz) potatoes and unlimited other vegetables, mint sauce and low-fat gravy

9 Baked trout with smoked garlic and pesto topping (page 181) served with 115g (4oz) new potatoes plus a large salad

10 Hot pan smoked salmon (page 184) served with 115g (4oz) new potatoes plus 300g (10oz) other seasonal vegetables

11 Griddled lamb's liver with tomato and bacon salsa (page 93) served with 115g (4oz) new potatoes and salad

12 (V) Lentil and roast vegetable loaf (page 132) served with 1 medium (approximately 180g) jacket potato

13 (V) Leek and sundried tomato risotto (page 140) served with 75g (3oz) French bread and a green salad

14 Chicken spaghetti (page 138) served with 75g (3oz) French bread and green salad

PUDDINGS

Here is a selection of puddings which you may or may not choose to include in your everyday eating plan. Some are as quick as just a couple of pieces of fresh fruit, or a branded readymade pudding, or you can make one of the delicious recipes included in this book. Any of these would grace a dinner party or could be offered as a treat for the family.

All these puddings are low in fat and so do not need to be included in your treat allowance unless you have no other calories to play with.

100-calorie puddings

1 (V) Fresh fruit salad verde (page 149)

2 (V) 1 meringue nest topped with 25g (1oz) any fresh fruit and 1 tablespoon low-fat yogurt

3 (V) 2 scoops fruit sorbet

4 1 × 150g pot low-fat yogurt or fromage frais (maximum 100 kcal)

5 Raspberry bavarois (page 154)

6 (V) 150g Total 0% fat Greek yogurt mixed with 1 level teaspoon runny honey

7 (V) Mango and white rum ice (page 147)

8 (V) Chestnut meringue roulade (page 148)

9　Orange Panna Cotta with fresh orange (page 153)

10　(V) Kiwi and passion fruit salad with balsamic dressing (page 156)

150-calorie puddings

1　(V) Lime cheesecake ice cream (page 150)

2　(V) Cinnamon and lemon prunes with saffron fromage frais (page 146)

3　(V) Burgundy poached peaches with strawberry salsa (page 152)

4　(V) 225g (8oz) strawberries topped with 115g (4oz) Wall's 'Too Good to be True' iced dessert

5　(V) 2 × 150g pots low-fat yogurt (maximum 150 kcal in total)

6　(V) 175g (6oz) fresh fruit salad topped with 1 × 150g low-fat yogurt (maximum 100 kcal)

7　(V) 1 meringue nest filled with 50g (2oz) fresh fruit plus 2 tablespoons low-fat yogurt or fromage frais

8　1 × 125g pot ready-to-eat raspberry flavour jelly topped with 175g (6oz) fresh raspberries

9　(V) 150ml (¼ pint) instant custard made with semi-skimmed milk plus ½ a small chopped banana

10　(V) 75g (3oz) dried apricots

TREATS

Here is a selection of treats from which you may choose each day, or save up for a bigger one. Some are low fat (less than 4% fat) and some are high fat. The choice is yours. Don't feel guilty if you want to select from the high-fat ones. Have your treat and enjoy it but then stop. If you find that having a taste of chocolate sets you off on a chocolate binge, then don't tempt yourself again for the moment. In time you may be able to be satisfied with small amounts and find you *can* be trusted. Only you can know when you reach this healthy balance of a relaxed attitude to those foods that once controlled you. But please be assured it can be done. I've been there. I know! My passion for ice cream is well known but now I can keep tubs of Häagen-Dazs in the freezer and only eat it on special occasions. It has no hold over me any more. And when I do have some, it is just a scoop, not the whole tub!

If you know there is a food type that you just adore, acknowledge it to yourself. The last thing you should do is pretend that it isn't tempting! Avoid keeping it in the house until you think you can be trusted and when you do, only buy one (don't stock up) to limit your likely downfall. Only eat it *with* someone so that second and third helpings are more difficult. Savour the flavour and appreciate it. Once you've had it, forget about it and move on to do something that takes your mind off food. Then give yourself a great big pat on the back if you get to the end of the day without giving into temptation.

Remember it's fear that you won't be able to control your eating of it that makes your consciousness towards the 'treat' much more acute. Try to chill out about it. Yes you can have more – another day. This is not your last chance to eat it. Tomorrow it is not going to be declared a 'banned substance'! Relax!

150 calories (4% or less fat)

50g (2oz) seedless raisins

8 sponge fingers

50g (2oz) slice malt loaf

6 Trebor barley sugars

10 Liquorice Allsorts

1 packet fruit gums

115g (4oz) oven chips

3 Matteson's turkey rashers, grilled and served on 1 medium slice wholemeal bread

1 × 150g pot low-fat custard plus ½ small chopped banana

150 calories (more than 4% fat)

30g bag potato hoops

39g Cadbury's Crème Egg

1 snack size Picnic

2 treat size bags Cadbury's Chocolate Buttons

1 Dime bar

5 chocolate orange éclair sweets

2 Wispa treat size bars

25g (1oz) Bombay Mix

4 Cadbury's Roses chocolates

25g bag ready salted crisps

10 Peardrop sweets

200 calories (more than 4% fat)

25g (1oz) butter

1 onion bhaji

1 small avocado

2 level tablespoons mayonnaise

30g (1¼oz) Bombay Mix

50g (2oz) Parmesan cheese

250 calories (more than 4% fat)

25ml (1fl oz) oil (all varieties)

1 vegetable samosa

50ml (2fl oz) double cream

30ml (1½fl oz) clotted cream

50g (2oz) taramasalata

300 calories (more than 4% fat)

3 large chocolate Digestive biscuits

4 Ferrero Rocher chocolates

1 Bounty bar

65g size Mars bar

61g Snickers bar

6 McDonald's Chicken McNuggets

1 chip shop cod in batter

49g bar Cadbury's Dairy Milk

49g bar Cadbury's Wholenut

60g bag Skittles

450 calories (more than 4% fat)

85g bar Galaxy

100g Mars bar

1 McDonald's milk shake

115g (4oz) After Eight mints

115g (4oz) Quality Street chocolates

115g (4oz) Cheddar cheese

1 Sharwoods Pot Noodle (Chinese curry flavour)

9 McDonald's Chicken McNuggets
1 McDonald's Quarter Pounder
1 portion McDonald's Large Fries

Fat and calorie content of foods

Here are some at-a-glance calorie calculations to help you plan your meals.

	Per 100g	
	Kcal	Fat (%)
Meat products		
Beefburgers	265	20.5
Black pudding	305	21.9
Corned beef	217	12.1
Cornish pasty	332	20.4
Faggots	268	18.5
Haggis	310	21.7
Luncheon meat	313	26.9
Meat paste	173	11.2
Pâté	316	28.9
Pork pie	376	27.0
Salami	491	45.2
Sausage roll	477	36.4
Sausages	299	24.1
Steak and kidney pie	323	21.2
Stewed steak (canned)	176	12.5
Bolognese sauce	145	11.1
Moussaka	184	13.6
Shepherd's pie	118	6.2
White fish		
Cod	76	0.7
Haddock	73	0.6

	Per 100g	
	Kcal	Fat (%)
Halibut	92	2.4
Lemon sole	81	1.4
Plaice	91	2.2
Whiting	92	0.9
Fatty fish		
Anchovies	280	19.9
Herring	234	18.5
Kipper	205	11.4
Mackerel	223	16.3
Pilchards	126	5.4
Salmon	182	12.0
Sardines	177	11.6
Trout	135	4.5
Tuna in brine	99	0.6
Tuna in oil	189	9.0
Whitebait (fried)	525	47.5
Crab	127	5.2
Lobster	119	3.4
Prawns	107	1.8
Scampi	316	17.6
Shrimps	73	0.8
Cockles	48	0.3
Mussels	87	2.0
Squid	66	1.5
Fish cakes	188	10.5
Fish fingers	233	12.7
Fish paste	169	10.4
Fish pie	105	3.0
Kedgeree	166	7.9
Roe	202	11.9
Taramasalata	446	46.4

	Per 100g				Per 100g	
	Kcal	Fat (%)			Kcal	Fat (%)
Fruit				Peaches	33	0.1
Apples	47	0.1		Paw paw	36	0.1
Apricots: fresh	31	0.1		Pears	40	0.1
dried	158	0.6		Pineapple	41	0.2
Avocado	190	19.5		Plums	36	0.1
Bananas	95	0.3		Prunes	79	0.2
Blackberries	25	0.2		Raisins	272	0.4
Blackcurrants	28	Tr		Raspberries	25	0.3
Cherries	48	0.1		Rhubarb	7	0.1
Clementines	37	0.1		Satsumas	36	0.1
Currants	267	0.4		Strawberries	27	0.1
Damsons	34	Tr		Sultanas	275	0.4
Dates	227	0.2		Tangerines	35	0.1
Figs	209	1.5				
Gooseberries	19	0.4		**Vegetables**		
Grapefruit	30	0.1		Asparagus	25	0.6
Grapes	60	0.1		Aubergine	15	0.4
Kiwi	49	0.5		Baked Beans	84	0.6
Lemons	19	0.3		Beans: green	24	0.5
Lychees	58	0.1		broad	81	0.6
Mandarins (canned in juice)	32	Tr		red kidney	103	0.5
Mangoes	57	0.2		butter	77	0.5
Melon: cantaloupe	19	0.1		runner	22	0.4
honeydew	28	0.1		Beetroot (raw)	36	0.1
watermelon	31	0.3		Broccoli	33	0.9
Mixed peel	231	0.9		Brussels sprouts	42	1.4
Nectarines	40	0.1		Beansprouts	31	0.5
Olives	103	11.0		Cabbage	26	0.4
Oranges	37	0.1		Carrots	35	0.3
Passion fruit	36	0.4		Cauliflower	34	0.9

	Per 100g	
	Kcal	Fat (%)
Celery	7	0.2
Chicory	11	0.6
Courgettes	18	0.4
Cucumber	10	0.1
Curly kale	33	1.6
Fennel	12	0.2
Leeks	22	0.5
Lettuce	14	0.5
Marrow	12	0.2
Mushrooms	13	0.5
Okra	31	1.0
Potatoes	75	0.2
Onions	36	0.2
Parsnips	66	1.2
Peas	83	1.5
Peas: mange tout	32	0.2
Peppers	20	0.6
Pumpkin	13	0.2
Quorn	86	3.5
Radish	12	0.2
Runner beans	22	0.4
Spinach	25	0.8
Spring greens	33	1.0
Spring onions	23	0.5
Swede	24	0.3
Sweetcorn (canned)	23	0.4
Tomatoes	17	0.3
Turnips	23	0.3
Watercress	22	1.0

ALCOHOL

	Kcal
Beer 300ml ($\frac{1}{2}$ pint)	90
Cider 300ml ($\frac{1}{2}$ pint)	100
Cider vintage 300ml ($\frac{1}{2}$ pint)	280
Lager 300ml ($\frac{1}{2}$ pint)	90
Spirits: 1 pub measure	50
Wine: 150ml (5fl oz)	
Dry white	95
Sparkling	110
Rosé	100
Red	100

Non-alcoholic drinks

	Kcal
Fruit juice: 150ml (5fl oz)	
Apple	50
Grape	75
Grapefruit	50
Orange	50
Pineapple	70
Tomato	30
Squashes: 25ml (1fl oz)	
undiluted	30
Mixers: 120ml (4fl oz)	
Ginger ale	40
Bitter lemon	50
Dry ginger	25
Tonic water	35
Lemonade	30
Fizzy drinks: 330ml can	
Cola	130
Ginger beer	100
Lemonade	80

Motivation: finding the willpower

I am often asked how it's possible to drum up the willpower to stick to a diet and exercise regime. My experience shows that if you have a good enough reason for wanting to lose weight, you can definitely do it. Imagine if someone were to offer you £50,000 if you could lose all your excess weight by a certain date. Do you think you could do it? Yes, of course you could. Why? Because the reward would be great enough to inspire you to make the effort and put into practice all that was needed to achieve your goal. You'd pull out all the stops to ensure that nothing got in your way to make you to stray off course. Motivation and having a positive mental attitude are crucial to the success of your diet and fitness campaign, as indeed they are in any aspect of life. Those people who just drift through life tend to get nowhere. It is the ones who have the motivation to succeed who become the great achievers.

Here are my top ten tips to help you get in the right frame of mind. Take these on board, and you will be well on the way to becoming a great achiever.

Set yourself some goals

If you want to lose weight and get fit you need to have some goals. In this instance I am not talking about losing a set amount of inches or being able to get into a size 10, but a goal that provides a deadline for you to work towards and a reason for losing as much weight as possible by that date. Be realistic – don't expect to lose four stone in two months – but your goal should provide a sufficient challenge so that you have to concentrate your mind and energy to achieve it. Decide to join your local Rosemary Conley Diet and Fitness class, join a running or walking club, tennis club, dance class. Include some short-term and some long-term goals. Write them down.

As you achieve your first goal tick it off. Then you need to set another goal to *keep* you motivated. Even if you've already achieved your target weight, you still need an incentive to encourage you to stay at that weight.

Reward yourself

As you achieve each goal, it's important that you reward yourself. It may be sufficient to be able to look stunning in a new outfit at a wedding or special celebration but that is pretty short term. If you don't have a specific event to attend, then reward yourself with a day at a health spa, a meal out with your partner or friend, or treat yourself to a new outfit. You need to give yourself an enjoyable 'pat on the back' for making the effort. We deserve self-care time and we deserve reward for our efforts. And to remind yourself of what you have achieved, place tins or packets of food of an equivalent weight that you have lost in a carrier bag and keep it in your wardrobe. Pick it up often to remind yourself of your progress. Realise that you used to carry that weight around with you all the time – and now you don't.

Stop making excuses

There'll never be a week or month when there isn't a birthday, a special meal out, or a million and one other reasons why it isn't a good time to start a diet. Stop making excuses – I think I've heard them all – and get on with the job in hand. If you want to lose weight and get fit, you can. Only you can do it, but you have to want to do it badly enough.

Be realistic

Just as we cannot change our height or our genes, neither can we change our bone structure or our basic physiological shape. But there is an enormous amount we can do to improve the way we look. As well as losing weight, set yourself a goal to restyle your hair, maybe colour it. Have a 'colour analysis' so you only buy clothes in colours that suit you. Remember, too, that healthy eating and regular exercise can make us glow with health, tone us up as we slim down and give us a greater sense of wellbeing. Truly, you *can* transform yourself yet still be realistic.

Record your progress

It's so easy to forget what we looked like at our heaviest, so before you start your diet and fitness campaign, ask someone to take a couple of photographs of you – a front view and a side view. Next, find yourself a pair of tight-fitting trousers or a skirt and set this garment aside as your measuring tool. Try it on every few days so that you have tangible proof of how many inches you are actually losing. Often, we don't realise how much progress we are actually making and we need a constant reminder of our achievements.

Develop the habit of enthusiasm

Be enthusiastic and focus on the many benefits you will be enjoying within days of starting your diet and fitness campaign. Make a note in your diary of all the good things you feel about yourself. As your whole attitude towards yourself and your body changes your self-esteem will increase.

Remove temptation

It is essential that you remove temptation from your kitchen and place of work. If you must have any sort of high-fat foods in the house – chocolate, biscuits, crisps and so on – keep them stored away in a place that is difficult to reach or under lock and key. If the food isn't there, you won't miss it, but if it is staring you in the face every time you open the cupboard, you will find it very difficult to resist.

Learn to cope with the difficult times

No matter how determined and conscientious you may be, there'll be occasions when your willpower weakens and your determination begins to flag. If you do have a minor indiscretion – or even a major one – don't think you've ruined all your hard work so far. You haven't. Just get right back on track, eat normal meals for the rest of the day and try to be more physically active to compensate. Do not skip meals ever!

Keep a scrapbook of your success

Buy yourself a scrapbook and make a note in it of all the good things that happen to you from now on. Fill it with photographs of yourself as you lose each stone or each time you do something new, something that you wouldn't have done when you were overweight. Looking back at this scrapbook on the 'bad' days could provide you with just the motivation you need to continue.

Picture yourself succeeding

Picture yourself wearing that beautiful dress or suit that you have had in your wardrobe for years but haven't been able to get into. Visualise yourself standing tall and slim, full of confidence, feeling really healthy and fit with lots of energy. If you want a better body, you can have one.

Honestly you can achieve it. Start today. What have you got to lose, except those unwanted pounds and inches?

Here are ten benefits you will enjoy if you lose weight and get fitter.

1 Clothes will fit!
Your clothes size will reduce faster than you think. Very soon you will feel so good wearing smaller clothes and you'll look great in them.

2 More energy!
You will have lots more energy. At the moment as you walk around it's as if you are carrying around a shopping bag or even a suitcase. Imagine how different it will feel when you have shed some of that weight. You will feel like you're dancing on air.

3 Your body will change!
Your body shape will improve dramatically. No matter whether you are heart shaped, apple shaped or pear shaped, as you lose weight your general shape will improve and your figure will become much more balanced. You will be amazed at how a low-fat eating plan can help you to change shape and look better than you ever dreamed you could.

4 Fashionable clothes!
You will be able to wear more fashionable clothes and look terrific. Trendy outfits that you never dreamt you would be able to wear will look fabulous on you. Can you imagine how good you're going to feel when you walk into the fashion store and choose something off the smaller rail and every garment you try on looks great?

5 Your metabolic rate increases!
You can actually increase your metabolic rate through taking regular exercise, but it must be exercise that you enjoy. If you don't have fun exercising you are not going to carry on doing it, so it is crucial that you find a way of exercising that stimulates you. It can be going for a walk with the dog, playing football with the children, working out to one of my videos or going along to a fitness class. A combination of all of these is ideal as they all burn fat and all of them will make you fitter.

6 Feel fit! Feel healthy!
You will feel fitter and healthier. You will probably find that you don't have so many aches and pains. You will sleep better and will have more zest for life. It really is a win/win situation.

7 Stand by for compliments!
Be prepared to accept some compliments from your family and friends and when people comment that you've lost weight, try not to rebuff it and say: 'Well, I've still got a huge stomach or backside', or whatever. Try to acknowledge the compliment as a generous gift and appreciate it. Say: 'I'm glad you can see the

difference! I feel so much better now. Thank you!' You wouldn't like it if nobody commented, would you?

8 Confidence booster!

In a very short period of time you will find your self-confidence increasing greatly. You will find your whole attitude to life will improve and, amazingly, people won't irritate you so much! You will find you have more patience and your whole outlook on life will be a sunnier one. You may even find that you are better at doing your job. Even your relationship with your husband or partner and your children may improve. We just need to feel good about ourselves, and losing weight and getting fitter helps us achieve that.

9 Do your family a favour!

Don't feel that you have to cook special food just for you and give the family other foods. A healthy, low-fat diet is suitable for everyone, though very young children can be given additional foods that contain more fat, such as cheese, eggs and even a little butter.

10 Look ten years younger!

Without doubt, one of the things that I have noticed when we photograph the successful slimmers for my magazine is that they all look years younger than when they were overweight. Being overweight does make us look older, so if you want to look younger, lose those excesses. You'll be so glad you did. Teaching everyone

healthy eating habits now will change their lives and their family's lives in the future. It is probably the best gift you could give them and, remember, *nothing* tastes as good as being slim feels!

Keeping trim for good

When you reach your goal weight you will feel on top of the world, but the big challenge is yet to come – keeping that weight off for ever.

Hopefully, on this diet, you have not found it too difficult to eat healthily yet enjoyably. The key now is to still keep to the low-fat way of cooking and eating. If you do, and you don't consciously *overeat*, then you shouldn't find maintaining your weight a problem. You will certainly find it easier if you keep up your activity levels and also refrain from nibbling between meals.

However, it is important that you eat more now than you did when you were trying to lose weight and you can be more relaxed with regard to carefully looking at the fat content of every food you buy. But beware the slippery slope of getting the taste for fat back again. Having a little butter on that bread roll in a restaurant, a little cream on your dessert, and chips more than occasionally can find you right back where you started. Just picture yourself as you felt then. Remember what you felt like, how tired you were all the time, how you never felt good in your clothes, how much older you looked, how much higher your blood pressure and/or cholesterol used to be. Don't go back there. You've done the hard work, don't throw it away now.

You know from the tables on pages 19–20 how many calories you need to eat to lose weight. When you reach your goal weight you need to gradually increase this total, initially by 200 calories daily and then a further 100 calories until you have increased your daily intake by around 600–800 calories, depending how physically active you are..

You may be thinking 'If I ate that much I know I will gain weight'. The fact is that most of us eat more calories than we think we do. So, in short, proceed with caution and you should be able to find the right level for you.

If you find you want to eat more, then just balance it with increased physical activity. Given time, your body (and your clothes) will tell you that your weight is either staying constant or increasing. I rarely weigh myself now – perhaps three or four times a year – as I know from the mirror and my clothes how I'm doing.

At our Rosemary Conley Diet and Fitness Clubs we do not pressurise the members who have reached their goal to weigh in every week. We suggest once a month is quite sufficient. What is so great about our classes is that whether you are aiming to lose weight or have reached your goal and are just maintaining your target weight, the exercise session included in the classes helps members burn fat and calories as well as keeping them fit and toned.

Some of the members in my own classes have been joining me every Monday night in Leicester for over 20 years! They have better, trimmer figures and much healthier bodies as a result. If I had been running a 'slimming only' club they would not have kept coming and would no doubt be much heavier and less healthy as a result.

So, keep up the good habits learnt within this or any of my earlier books. Keep as active as you can – any and every bit of activity will help to keep you slim.

Soups

The foundation of good soup lies in having fresh core ingredients coupled with a good flavoursome stock. These days, fresh stocks are readily available, along with bouillon stock powder, which simplifies the seasoning of soups and sauces. This instant powder can be sprinkled into the dish during cooking or at the finish, allowing total control over flavouring.

Soup has many forms, from clear crisp consommés garnished with baby vegetables or grains such as pearl barley, to others that are roux based, thickened with flour; a more substantial preparation is to purée, giving a rich, thick, velvety consistency.

Some of the recipes call for a little low-fat fromage frais stirred in just prior to serving. Low-fat Normandy fromage frais (available from most supermarkets) is preferable, as it is smoother than other brands. This adds a rich, creamy effect. Always use this as the finishing touch, as otherwise it may cause the soup to curdle if it is reboiled.

Simple tomato and roasted garlic soup

This soup requires forward thinking. The garlic needs to be roasted for approximately 45 minutes before you make the soup. Roasting the garlic gives it a much mellower flavour than usual, so it's a good idea to roast a couple of whole heads together while you have the oven on. Wrapped in foil, it will keep in the refrigerator for up to one week. It makes a good substitute for smoked garlic.

1 Preheat the oven to 200C, 400F, Gas Mark 6.
2 Remove the outer skin from the garlic bulb and slice the top off. Place in a square piece of foil and wrap around to form a parcel.
3 Place in the oven for 45 minutes until soft. Remove from the oven and allow to cool.
4 Pour the canned tomatoes into a liquidiser or food processor and purée until smooth.
5 Squeeze out the garlic purée from the roasted bulb and add to the food processor.
6 Push the mixture through a sieve into a saucepan to remove the tomato seeds. Add the spring onions and the vegetable stock with sufficient water to give a good consistency and bring to the boil. Stir in the basil.
7 Season to taste with salt and pepper and serve.

SERVES 4
PER SERVING:
62 KCAL/0.7G FAT
PREPARATION TIME:
5 MINUTES
COOKING TIME:
50 MINUTES

1 whole head garlic
3 × 400g (3 × 14oz) cans plum tomatoes
6 spring onions, finely chopped
3 teaspoons vegetable bouillon stock powder
1 tablespoon chopped fresh basil
salt and freshly ground black pepper

Black bean and smoked bacon soup

SERVES 6
PER SERVING:
182 KCAL/5G FAT
PREPARATION TIME:
20 MINUTES
COOKING TIME:
40–45 MINUTES

175g (6oz) black beans, soaked
overnight
2 medium onions, finely
chopped
2 carrots, finely diced
1 celery stick, finely diced
2 garlic cloves, crushed
1 teaspoon ground coriander
1.2 litres (2 pints) vegetable
stock
1 tablespoon chopped fresh
marjoram
2 bay leaves
115g (4oz) lean smoked bacon,
finely chopped
salt and freshly ground black
pepper
4 tomatoes, peeled, seeded and
finely chopped to garnish
2 tablespoons chopped fresh
coriander to garnish

Serve this soup as a wholesome lunch or liquidise and serve as an evening soup flavoured with a little Madeira wine.

IMPORTANT: Black beans should always be soaked overnight and boiled rapidly for at least 10 minutes at the start of cooking. Do not eat uncooked beans.

1 After soaking overnight, rinse the black beans well in plenty of cold running water and place in a large saucepan with the onions, carrots, celery, garlic, ground coriander and stock.
2 Bring to the boil, and boil rapidly for 10 minutes, then reduce the heat to a gentle simmer, add the marjoram, bay leaves and smoked bacon. Cover and simmer gently for 40–45 minutes until the beans are soft.
3 Season to taste with salt and pepper and adjust the consistency, adding more stock if required.
4 Ladle into warmed serving bowls and garnish with the chopped tomato and fresh coriander.

Cream of asparagus soup

Asparagus can be bought in many different grades from thick jumbo stems to the thin fine spear. Choose a thick to medium thickness of stem, as the finer stems will disintegrate when cooked over this length of time.

1 Prepare the asparagus by trimming away the stalk at the point where the stem breaks when snapped in half. Trim off the tips and reserve. Chop the remaining stems into small pieces.
2 In a non-stick pan dry-fry the onions until soft. Add the garlic and thyme and continue cooking for 1–2 minutes. Add 3 tablespoons of vegetable stock, then sprinkle the flour over and cook out for 1 minute, stirring well with a wooden spoon.
3 Gradually add the remaining stock along with the skimmed milk and asparagus stems. Add the bay leaves and gently simmer for 15–20 minutes until the asparagus is just cooked and the soup has slightly thickened.
4 Five minutes before serving stir in the asparagus tips and season to taste.
5 Serve piping hot garnished with chopped chives.

SERVES 4
PER SERVING:
105 KCAL/1.3G FAT
PREPARATION TIME:
10 MINUTES
COOKING TIME:
30–35 MINUTES

225g (8oz) fresh asparagus
2 medium onions, finely chopped
2 garlic cloves, crushed
1 teaspoon chopped fresh thyme
450ml (¾ pint) vegetable stock
1 tablespoon plain flour
450ml (¾ pint) skimmed milk
2 bay leaves
salt and freshly ground black pepper
1 tablespoon chopped fresh chives to garnish

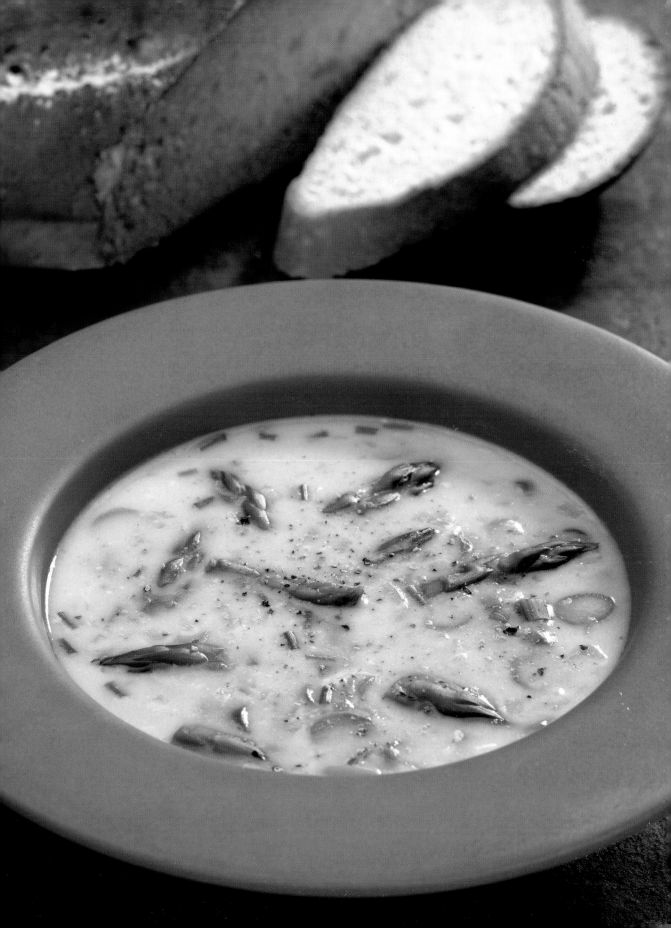

Cream of leek and wild mushroom soup

Be selective when buying dried mushrooms. Check for good-sized pieces, not broken or shrivelled dark flakes, as these can be hard and chewy when reconstituted. Adding a little lemon zest to the soup really enhances the strong mushroom flavours.

1. Place the mushrooms, garlic, thyme and stock into a small saucepan and gently simmer for 10 minutes in order to soften the mushrooms.
2. In a separate non-stick pan dry-fry the leeks until soft. Add the lemon zest with 3 tablespoons of the mushroom stock.
3. Sprinkle the flour over and cook out for 1 minute, stirring well with a wooden spoon.
4. Gradually add the mushroom stock and the contents of the saucepan along with the skimmed milk. Add the bay leaves and gently simmer for 20–25 minutes until the mushrooms are soft and the soup has slightly thickened.
5. Just before serving, stir in the chopped parsley and season to taste.
6. Serve with crusty bread.

SERVES 4
PER SERVING:
91 KCAL / 1.6G FAT
PREPARATION TIME:
10 MINUTES
COOKING TIME:
35–40 MINUTES

40g (1 ½oz) good quality dried wild mushrooms
2 garlic cloves, crushed
1 teaspoon chopped fresh thyme
450ml (¾ pint) vegetable stock
4–5 young leeks, finely chopped
1 teaspoon finely grated lemon zest
1 tablespoon plain flour
450ml (¾ pint) skimmed milk
2 bay leaves
1 tablespoon chopped fresh parsley
salt and freshly ground black pepper

Courgette and basil soup

SERVES 4
PER SERVING:
102 KCAL/1.7G FAT
PREPARATION TIME:
10 MINUTES
COOKING TIME:
30 MINUTES

1kg (2lb) young courgettes
2 medium onions, chopped
2 garlic cloves, crushed
600ml (1 pint) vegetable stock
1 teaspoon fresh thyme leaves
2 bay leaves
300ml ($\frac{1}{2}$ pint) skimmed milk
salt and freshly ground black
    pepper
20 fresh basil leaves to garnish

Always select small young courgettes with a brightly coloured skin free from wrinkles. Aged courgettes can taste bitter and sour. Make the soup in advance and store chilled until required.

1 Top and tail the courgettes and roughly chop.
2 Place in a large saucepan with the remaining ingredients except the skimmed milk and basil. Bring to the boil, then reduce the heat and simmer gently for 15–20 minutes until the vegetables are soft.
3 Allow to cool slightly, then liquidise in batches, adding a little of the milk and basil to each batch until smooth and lump free. Return to the pan and season to taste.
4 Adjust the consistency with a little extra milk if required, garnish with finely shredded basil leaves and serve immediately.

Sweetcorn and red pepper soup

An easy colourful soup to brighten up your day. Most of the ingredients can be stored in your food cupboard, making it a quick and easy lunch for all the family.

1 In a large non-stick pan dry-fry the shallots until soft.
2 Sprinkle the paprika over, add the garlic and cook for 2–3 minutes, stirring well. Add the peppers, corn and chilli and stir in the stock. Bring to the boil, then reduce the heat to a gentle simmer.
3 Slake the cornflour with a little cold water and add to the soup, stirring well to prevent any lumps forming. Cook for 5–6 minutes until the soup thickens slightly.
4 Serve garnished with chopped chives.

SERVES 4
PER SERVING:
50 KCAL/1.1G FAT
PREPARATION TIME:
10 MINUTES
COOKING TIME:
20 MINUTES

4 small shallots, finely chopped
1 teaspoon paprika
2 smoked garlic cloves, crushed
2 red peppers, finely diced
1 × 175g (6oz) can sweetcorn, drained
pinch of dried chilli flakes
600ml (1 pint) vegetable stock
2 teaspoons cornflour
1 tablespoon finely chopped chives to garnish

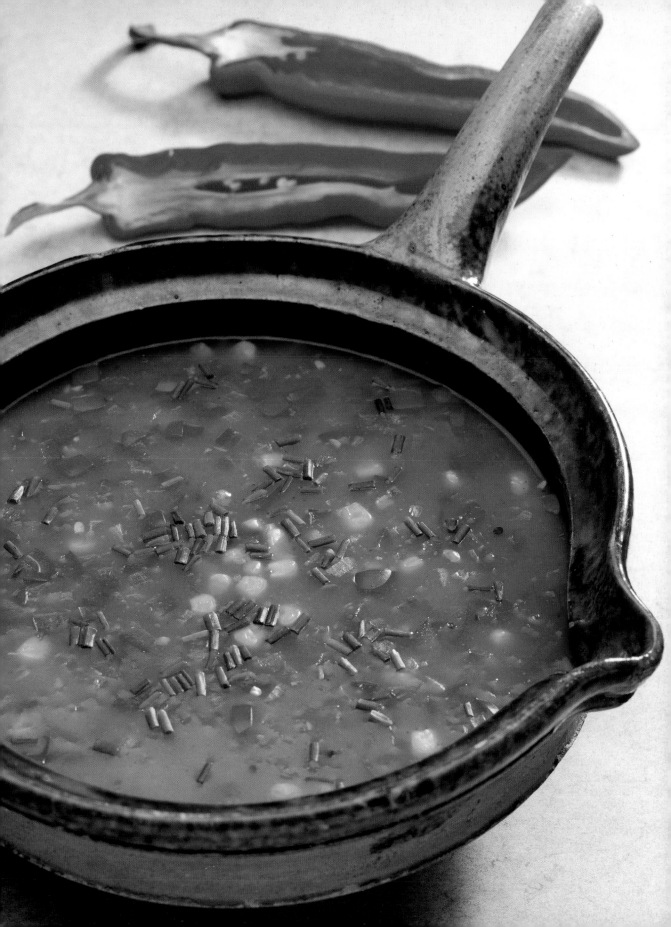

Parsnip and apple soup with Calvados

A classic combination of sweet and sour. The flaming Calvados adds a finishing touch to this delightful, comforting soup.

1 Peel and slice the parsnips, place in a saucepan with the celery, onions and garlic and dry-fry over a low heat for 2–3 minutes.
2 Peel, core and slice the apples. Add them, the thyme, stock and bay leaves and simmer gently until the vegetables are soft. Remove the bay leaves and liquidise until smooth.
3 Return the soup to the pan, adjust the consistency with a little extra stock if required and season with salt and black pepper.
4 Just before serving, remove from the heat and stir in the fromage frais.
5 Divide into serving bowls. Heat the Calvados in a metal ladle over a low heat, then ignite with a long match. Pour the flaming brandy over the soup and serve.

SERVES 4
PER SERVING:
249 KCAL/3.4G FAT
PREPARATION TIME:
20 MINUTES
COOKING TIME:
30 MINUTES

1 kg (2lb) fresh young parsnips
3 celery sticks, sliced
2 medium onions, chopped
1 garlic clove, crushed
2 large Bramley cooking apples
2 teaspoons chopped fresh thyme
1.2 litres (2 pints) vegetable stock
2 bay leaves
2 tablespoons virtually fat free fromage frais
2 tablespoons Calvados brandy
salt and freshly ground black pepper

Watercress and potato soup

SERVES 4
PER SERVING:
138 KCAL/1G FAT
PREPARATION TIME:
10 MINUTES
COOKING TIME:
20 MINUTES

4 baby leeks, finely sliced

2 garlic cloves, crushed

3 baking potatoes, peeled and
    diced

1.2 litres (2 pints) vegetable
    stock bouillon

1 tablespoon plain flour

1/2 teaspoon ground mace

1 tablespoon finely chopped
    fresh marjoram

1 bunch watercress, tops
    removed

salt and freshly ground black
    pepper

a little low-fat fromage frais to
    garnish

Ground mace is the outer husk of the spice nutmeg. It has a very unusual flavour, but use sparingly, as too much may result in a strong bitter aftertaste.

1 In a non-stick pan dry-fry the baby leeks and garlic for 2–3 minutes over a moderate heat, until softened but not coloured.

2 Add the potatoes and 3 tablespoons of stock and stir in the flour and the ground mace. Cook over a low heat, stirring well, for 1 minute in order to cook out the flour.

3 Gradually add the remaining stock, stirring well to prevent any lumps forming. Add the marjoram and bring to the boil, then reduce the heat and simmer for 20 minutes.

4 Just before serving, season to taste with salt and black pepper and add the watercress. Pour into a warmed serving tureen and garnish with a little low-fat fromage frais.

Spring vegetable soup

A celebration of fresh new spring vegetables. Make the soup in advance and reheat as required, adding the spring greens just at the end to prevent them overcooking.

1 In a non-stick pan dry-fry the baby leeks, carrots and courgettes for 2–3 minutes over a moderate heat, until softened but not coloured.
2 Stir in the stock and chopped tomatoes.
3 Slake the cornflour with a little water and stir into the soup, bringing the soup up to the boil. Reduce the heat and simmer gently for 10–15 minutes.
4 Five minutes before serving, add the spring greens and season to taste with salt and black pepper. Serve immediately.

SERVES 4
PER SERVING:
69 KCAL/1.4G FAT
PREPARATION TIME:
10 MINUTES
COOKING TIME:
20 MINUTES
SUITABLE FOR FREEZING

4 baby leeks, finely sliced
2 small carrots, cut into thin strips
2 small courgettes, diced
1.2 litres (2 pints) vegetable stock bouillon
1 × 400g (14oz) can chopped tomatoes
2 teaspoons cornflour
2–3 leaves spring greens, finely chopped
salt and freshly ground black pepper

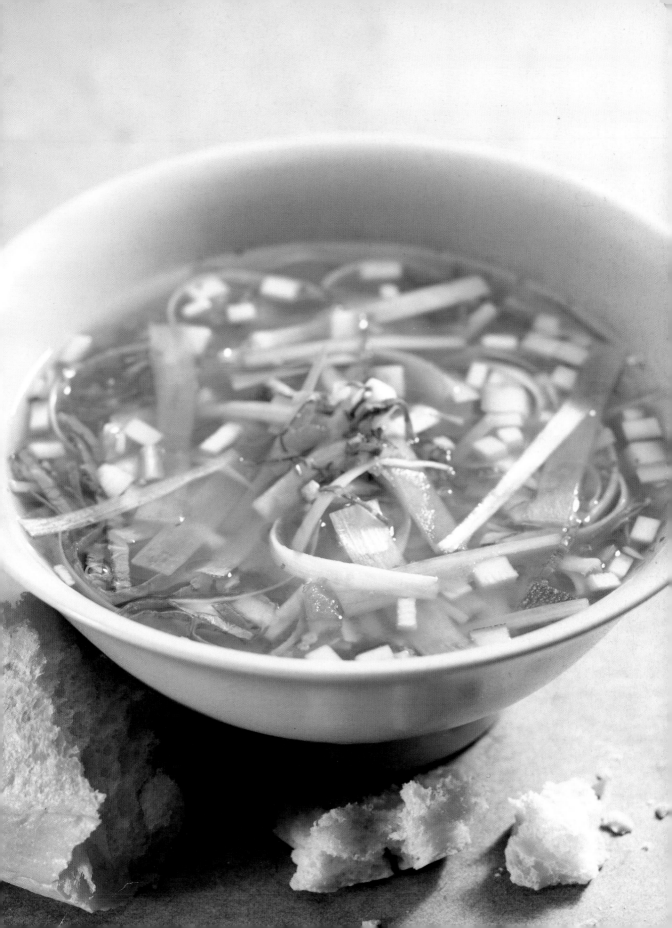

Spiced cauliflower soup

Cauliflower makes wonderful thick creamy soup. It is best to make it fresh and be sure not to re-boil the soup after it has been liquidised, as this may impair the flavour.

1 Remove and discard the outer leaves from the cauliflower and coarsely chop the rest, including the stalk. Place in a large saucepan with the remaining ingredients except the skimmed milk and fresh coriander. Bring to the boil, then reduce the heat and simmer gently for 15–20 minutes until the vegetables are soft.

2 Allow to cool slightly, then liquidise in batches, adding a little of the milk and coriander to each batch until smooth and lump free. Return to the pan and season to taste.

3 Adjust the consistency with a little extra milk if required, garnish with finely chopped coriander leaves and serve immediately.

SERVES 4
PER SERVING:
82 KCAL/1.4G FAT
PREPARATION TIME:
10 MINUTES
COOKING TIME:
30 MINUTES

1 large cauliflower
2 medium onions, chopped
2 smoked garlic cloves
600ml (1 pint) vegetable stock
2 teaspoons medium curry
   powder
1 teaspoon ground coriander
1 red chilli, finely chopped
300ml ($\frac{1}{2}$ pint) skimmed milk
2 tablespoons chopped fresh
   coriander
salt and freshly ground black
   pepper

Roasted shallot and spinach soup

SERVES 4
PER SERVING:
100 KCAL/1.6G FAT
PREPARATION TIME:
10 MINUTES
COOKING TIME:
40 MINUTES

450g (1lb) long shallots, peeled

300ml (½ pint) skimmed milk

2 garlic cloves, peeled and
    chopped

2 teaspoons fresh thyme

4 teaspoons cornflour

1 tablespoon Dijon mustard

225g (8oz) young baby leaf
    spinach

1.2 litres (2 pints) vegetable
    stock

salt and freshly ground black
    pepper

grated fresh nutmeg to garnish

Roasting the shallots releases their sweet natural juices, adding a distinctive roasted flavour to this flavoursome soup. If you are unable to get shallots, substitute baby leeks.

1 Preheat the oven to 200C, 400F, Gas Mark 6.
2 Slice the shallots in half and place on a non-stick baking tray. Season with salt and black pepper and roast in the top of the preheated oven for 20–25 minutes until soft.
3 Heat the milk, garlic and thyme in a medium-sized saucepan. Slake the cornflour with a little water and stir into the milk. Keep stirring as the sauce thickens, then reduce the heat and simmer for 2–3 minutes.
4 Stir in the mustard and spinach – if using large leaf spinach roughly chop first. Add half the stock along with the roasted shallots. Allow to cool.
5 When the mixture is quite cool, pour into a liquidiser and blend until smooth.
6 Return the soup to the pan, add the remaining stock and reheat.
7 Serve garnished with a little grated fresh nutmeg.

Celeriac and nutmeg soup

Celeriac is an unusual root vegetable with a distinctive nutty flavour – ideal for thick wholesome winter soups. It can also be boiled with potatoes to add flavour to mashed potatoes.

1. Dry-fry the onion and garlic in a non-stick saucepan until soft. Add the celeriac, thyme and stock. Simmer gently for 25–30 minutes until tender.
2. Pour the soup into a liquidiser or food processor and blend until smooth.
3. Return to the saucepan, adjusting the consistency with a little more stock or skimmed milk if required. Grate over a little fresh nutmeg and season with salt and black pepper.
4. Before serving, remove from the heat and stir in the fromage frais. Serve garnished with a sprig of parsley and a little grated fresh nutmeg.

SERVES 4
PER SERVING:
81 KCAL / 1.3G FAT
PREPARATION TIME:
15 MINUTES
COOKING TIME:
40 MINUTES

2 medium onions, chopped
2 garlic cloves, crushed
450g (1lb) celeriac, peeled and cut into chunks
1 tablespoon fresh thyme
1.2 litres (2 pints) vegetable stock
a little fresh nutmeg
salt and freshly ground black pepper
3 tablespoons low-fat fromage frais
flat leaf parsley to garnish

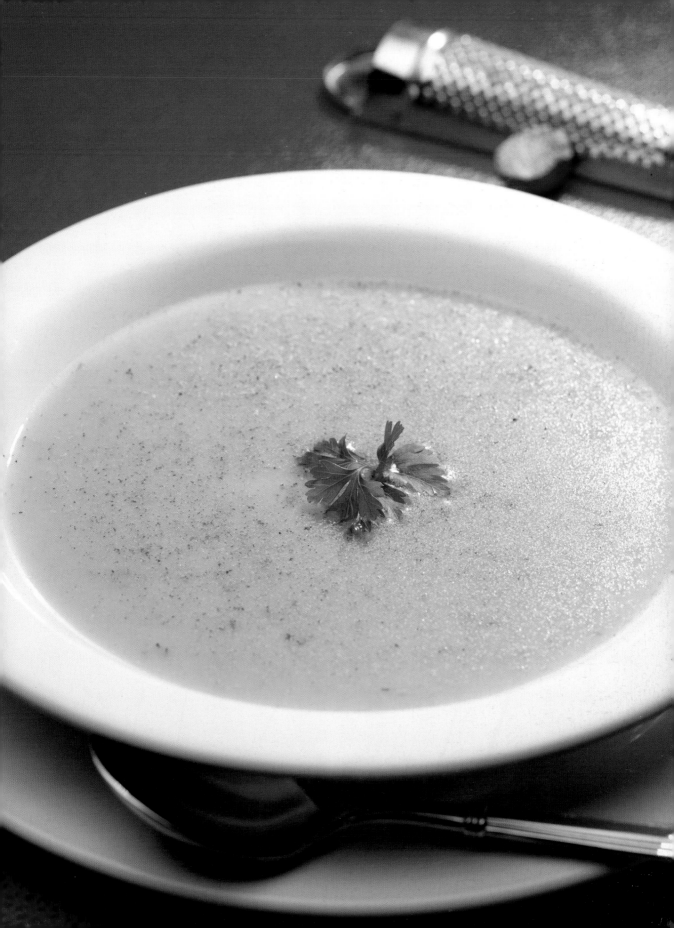

Potage paysanne

Cutting all the vegetables into similar-sized pieces adds style to a basic clear soup. Use fresh seasonal vegetables for maximum flavour.

1 Thinly slice all the root vegetables, and then cut them into small shapes, the size of a one-penny piece.
2 In a non-stick pan dry-fry the vegetables except the beans and peas for 2–3 minutes over a moderate heat, until softened but not coloured.
3 Stir in the stock and bring to the boil. Reduce the heat and simmer gently for 10–15 minutes.
4 Chop the beans into diagonal slices and add to the soup 10 minutes before serving, along with the peas.
5 Season to taste with salt and black pepper and stir in the chopped parsley.
6 Serve straight away with warm crusty bread.

SERVES 4
PER SERVING:
53 KCAL／1.6G FAT
PREPARATION TIME:
10 MINUTES
COOKING TIME:
20 MINUTES

4 baby leeks, finely sliced into small circles
2 small carrots
4 small turnips
2 sticks celery
6 spring onions
1.2 litres (2 pints) vegetable stock bouillon
50g (2oz) French green beans
50g (2oz) fresh peas
2 tablespoons chopped fresh parsley
salt and freshly ground black pepper

Minted green pea and cucumber soup

SERVES 4
PER SERVING:
104 KCAL/1.7G FAT
PREPARATION TIME:
10 MINUTES
COOKING TIME:
25 MINUTES

450g (1lb) frozen petit pois

1 medium onion, finely chopped

8 fresh mint leaves

1 young cucumber, peeled and chopped

600ml (1 pint) vegetable stock

1 tablespoon virtually fat free fromage frais

salt and freshly ground black pepper

Cucumber is a vegetable we tend to limit to salads and cold dishes. When cooked, it has a very delicate flavour. Try it in soups or simply stir-fried.

1 Place the peas and onion in a large saucepan, barely cover with salted water and boil for 20 minutes. Pour into a liquidiser or food processor and purée until smooth.

2 Add the mint and cucumber, along with the vegetable stock, and blend again until smooth. Return to the saucepan and reheat.

3 Season to taste with salt and pepper.

4 Just before serving, stir in the fromage frais.

Thai noodle soup

Bring the flavours of the orient to your table with this spicy wholesome soup. If you find you have to buy fresh spices such as lemongrass or ginger in large quantities, prepare them, then place in food bags and freeze for a later time.

1 In a large non-stick pan dry-fry the shallot until soft.
2 Crush the coriander seed on a chopping board with the broad side of a chopping knife and add to the pan. Add the garlic and cook for 2–3 minutes, then add the lemongrass, ginger, chilli, turmeric and stir well to combine the spices. Add the vegetable stock and bring to the boil. Reduce the heat to a gentle simmer and add the noodles.
3 Cook for 5–6 minutes until the noodles become soft, then remove from the heat and stir in the beansprouts and fromage frais.
4 Just before serving, garnish with mint leaves.

SERVES 1
PER SERVING:
175 KCAL/4.1G FAT
PREPARATION TIME:
20 MINUTES
COOKING TIME:
20 MINUTES

1 small shallot, finely sliced
$1/4$ teaspoon coriander seed
$1/2$ smoked garlic clove, crushed
$1/2$ teaspoon lemongrass, finely chopped
small piece fresh ginger, peeled and finely chopped
pinch of dried chilli flakes
pinch of ground turmeric
300ml ($1/2$ pint) vegetable stock
25g (1oz) [dry weight] egg noodles
25g (1oz) beansprouts
1 tablespoon virtually fat free Normandy fromage frais
mint leaves to garnish

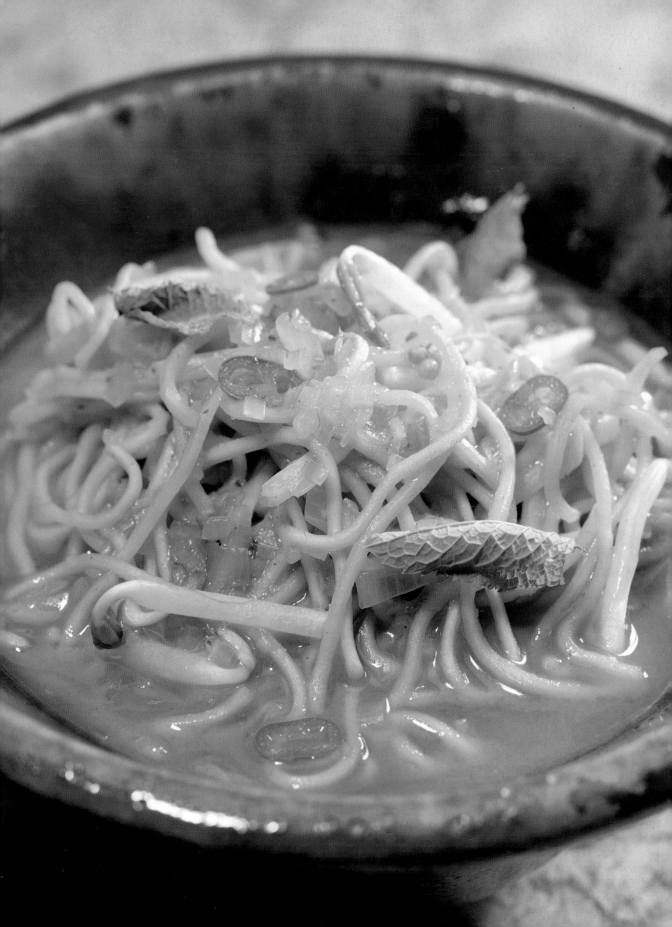

Meat and poultry

The selection of prepared meats available is endless and choosing the right cut can sometimes become quite daunting. Basic butchering can determine many factors, but the key rule is to choose clean, clear-coloured meat, not dull and grey in appearance and certainly without dried edges.

Small cuts should be evenly sliced or diced into uniform-sized pieces to ensure that they cook properly at the same time.

Organic or free range meat may seem slightly more expensive, but the compensation is well worth it in the form of both flavour and texture.

Meat should always be stored well-wrapped in the coldest part of the refrigerator. Most small cuts, including mince, are best used within 1–2 days of purchase. Generally red meat tends to keep better than white, but if in doubt – throw it out!

As with meat, the selection of poultry has expanded, offering farm-produced birds, again organically fed, or free range with a fuller flavour.

Supermarket birds are generally very lean, which can mean a compromise on flavour, so use marinades and stir-fry spices to pep them up. Proper chilled storage is imperative, as is making sure the poultry is completely cooked through.

Chilli beef enchiladas

SERVES 4
PER SERVING:
351 KCAL/13.4G FAT
(EXCLUDING TORTILLA)
PREPARATION TIME:
10 MINUTES
COOKING TIME:
35 MINUTES

450g (1lb) lean steak mince

2 medium onions, finely
  chopped

3 garlic cloves, crushed

2 beef stock cubes

1–2 fresh red chillies, chopped

2 red peppers, seeded and finely
  chopped

1 tablespoon chopped fresh
  oregano

1 × 400g (14oz) can chopped
  tomatoes

300ml (½ pint) tomato passata

300ml (½ pint) skimmed milk

3 teaspoons cornflour

4 Navajo Tortillas (see recipe,
  page 120)

50g (2oz) low-fat Cheddar
  cheese, grated

salt and freshly ground black
  pepper

Tortillas form the base to this Mexican feast. If you wish, replace the beef with minced chicken or pork, and a good vegetarian filling is roasted vegetables.

1 Preheat the oven to 200C, 400F, Gas Mark 6. In a preheated non-stick pan dry-fry the mince until lightly browned. Pour into a sieve to drain away the fat and wipe out the pan with kitchen paper.

2 Add the onions and garlic to the pan and dry-fry for 2–3 minutes until soft.

3 Return the meat to the pan and crumble the stock cubes over. Add the chillies, peppers, oregano and both the chopped and passata tomatoes. Simmer gently for 20–25 minutes until the sauce has thickened and the meat is tender.

4 In a separate pan heat the milk. Slake the cornflour with a little cold water and whisk into the milk. Stir as the sauce thickens, seasoning well with salt and freshly ground black pepper.

5 Take a tortilla and place a line of the beef mixture down the centre. Roll up and place in an ovenproof dish. Repeat with the remaining tortillas, placing any meat mix on top of each. Pour the sauce over and sprinkle with grated cheese.

6 Bake in the preheated oven for 20–25 minutes until golden brown. Serve with red pepper salsa and mixed green leaves.

Roast beef with Yorkshire pudding, dry-roast potatoes and parsnips

1 Preheat the oven to 180C, 350F, Gas Mark 4.

2 Prepare the beef by removing as much fat as possible. Place the onion, carrot, celery and herbs in the bottom of a roasting tin or ovenproof dish. Sit the beef on top and pour 300ml (½ pint) water around. Place in the oven. Allow 15 minutes per 450g (lb) plus 15 minutes for rare beef, 20 minutes per 450g (1lb) plus 20 minutes over for medium rare, and 25 minutes per 450g (1lb) plus 30 minutes if you like your beef well done.

3 Cook the potatoes and parsnips separately in boiling water. Drain and place in a non-stick roasting tin. Place in the top of the oven for 35–40 minutes until golden brown. You can baste the vegetables with the diluted soy sauce if they appear to dry out, depending on your oven.

4 Forty minutes before the beef is ready, make the Yorkshire pudding batter by blending the flour with the egg and a little milk to a smooth paste. Whisk in the remaining milk until smooth. Preheat a six-hole non-stick Yorkshire pudding tin for 2 minutes in the oven. Remove and half fill each mould with batter. Return to the oven and increase the heat to 200C, 400F, Gas Mark 6 for 35–40 minutes.

5 When the beef is cooked, remove from the tin and wrap in foil to keep warm. Allow to rest for 5–10 minutes. Meanwhile, add 600ml (1 pint) of beef stock to the pan juices. Slake the cornflour with a little water and add to the pan. Stir well as the gravy thickens. Add 1–2 drops of gravy browning as required.

6 To serve, carve the beef thinly and serve with Yorkshire pudding, dry–roast potatoes and parsnips, beef gravy and seasonal vegetables.

SERVES 6
PER SERVING:
BEEF: 218 KCAL/8.3G FAT
DRY-ROAST POTATOES AND PARSNIPS: 106 KCAL/0.9G FAT
YORKSHIRE PUDDING: 79 KCAL/1.3G FAT
PREPARATION TIME: 30 MINUTES
COOKING TIME: 1–1½ HOURS

1kg (2lb) joint lean beef, topside
1 onion, finely diced
1 carrot, diced
1 celery stick, diced
2 teaspoons mixed dried herbs
600ml (1 pint) beef stock
1 tablespoon cornflour
1–2 drops gravy browning

for the Yorkshire pudding batter
115g (4oz) plain flour
1 egg
pinch of salt
150ml (¼ pint) skimmed milk

for the dry-roast potatoes and parsnips
450g (1lb) potatoes, peeled and cut in half
8 medium parsnips, peeled and left whole
1 tablespoon soy sauce diluted in 2 tablespoons of water (optional)

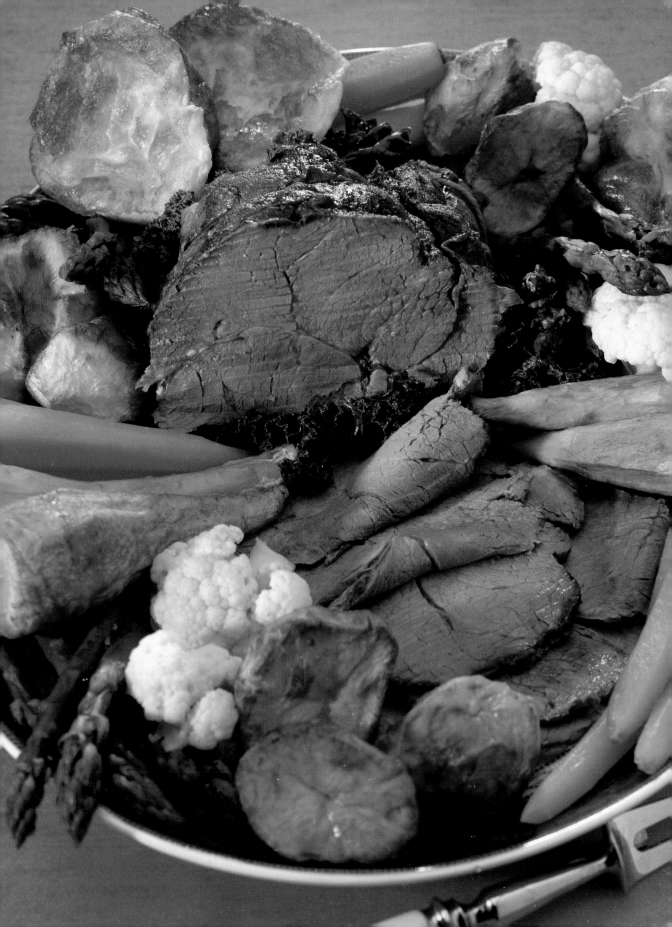

Steak and kidney pie

1 Preheat the oven to 180C, 350F, Gas Mark 4.

2 Trim the steak, removing all the fat, then cut the steak into cubes.

3 Preheat a non-stick frying pan. Dry-fry the cubes of beef steak and kidneys until well browned. Place in a 12 × 8in (30 × 20cm) pie dish. Dry-fry the onions until soft and add this to the meat in the pie dish.

4 Place 300ml (1/2 pint) water in the pan. Add the wine and stock cubes to the pan and bring to the boil. Mix the gravy powder with a little cold water and add to the boiling stock in the pan, stirring continuously. The gravy should be quite thick. Add more gravy powder mixed with a little water as necessary. Pour the gravy over the meat in the pie dish.

5 Boil the potatoes and drain. Mash the potatoes with the yogurt and sufficient skimmed milk to make the consistency quite soft. Season to taste.

6 Using a fork or a piping bag with a star nozzle, carefully spoon (or pipe) the 'creamed' potato on top of the meat and gravy and ensure that it covers it completely. If you spoon the potato on top, spread it carefully with a fork.

7 Place in the oven for 30–40 minutes, or until crisp and brown on top.

SERVES 4
PER SERVING:
355 KCAL / 6.8G FAT
PREPARATION TIME:
20 MINUTES
COOKING TIME:
50 MINUTES

225g (8oz) lean rump or sirloin steak, cut into cubes
225g (8oz) kidneys cut into bite-sized pieces
2 medium onions, chopped
1 wine glass red wine
2 beef stock cubes
1 tablespoon gravy powder
1kg (2lb) potatoes, peeled
2 tablespoons low-fat natural yogurt
4–5 tablespoons skimmed milk
salt and freshly ground black pepper

Serrano calf's liver

SERVES 4
PER SERVING:
184 KCAL/7G FAT
PREPARATION TIME:
30 MINUTES
COOKING TIME:
10 MINUTES

4 slices calf's liver

150ml (¼ pint) skimmed milk

1 teaspoon green peppercorns, crushed

4 thin slices Serrano ham

2 garlic cloves, crushed

300ml (½ pint) tomato passata

1 tablespoon mixed chopped fresh herbs (parsley, oregano, chives)

salt and freshly ground black pepper

Spain has long been a devotee of cured ham. The quality and flavour is determined by many factors, including the animal feed and curing process. Serrano ham is cured using only sea salt without the use of additives, resulting in lightly pink coloured meat with a sweet aroma and a firm texture.

1 Preheat the oven to 150C, 300F, Gas Mark 2.
2 Soak the liver in the milk for 30 minutes to clean the remove any bitter flavours.
3 Preheat a non-stick griddle pan. Add a little vegetable oil, then wipe out with kitchen paper.
4 Remove the liver from the milk and pat dry with kitchen paper. Season each piece on both sides with the green peppercorns and wrap individually with a slice of Serrano ham.
5 Cook the meat quickly in a hot pan for 2 minutes on each side. Remove and place in a warm oven while you make the sauce.
6 Add the garlic to the pan and cook quickly until soft. Pour in the passata, stirring well to pick up the pan juices. Add the herbs and season to taste with salt and freshly ground black pepper.

Red Thai beef

A quick hot and spicy beef dish that's packed full of flavour. Prepare the night before and leave covered overnight in the refrigerator for a tasty dinner accompanied with an exotic salad.

1 Remove any fat from the meat and discard. Slice the meat into thin strips and place into a shallow dish. Season well with salt and freshly ground black pepper.
2 Combine the remaining ingredients except the fresh coriander and pour over the beef. Leave to marinate for at least 1 hour, mixing periodically.
3 Strain the marinade from the beef and reserve. Preheat a non-stick frying pan and stir-fry the beef quickly over a high heat for 1–2 minutes until cooked to your liking. Add the reserved marinade and heat through.
4 Stir in the fresh coriander and serve on a bed of rice.

SERVES 4
PER SERVING:
169 KCAL/6G FAT
PREPARATION TIME:
10 MINUTES
COOKING TIME:
5 MINUTES

450g (1 lb) lean steak (rump or
　　sirloin)
1 beef stock cube dissolved in
　　150ml (1/4 pint) boiling water
4 tablespoons light soy sauce
1 teaspoon ground coriander
300ml (1/2 pint) tomato passata
1 small red chilli, finely sliced
1 teaspoon finely chopped
　　lemongrass
2 garlic cloves, crushed
1 tablespoon chopped fresh
　　coriander
salt and freshly ground black
　　pepper

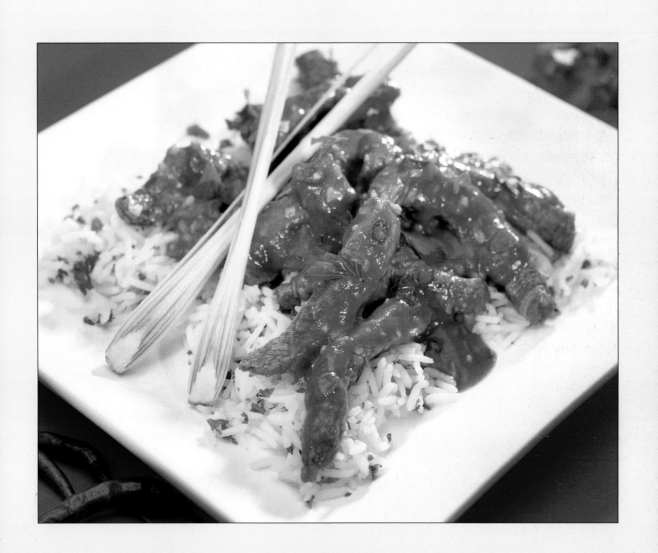

Tarragon pork

Tarragon is a primary herb with a strong distinctive flavour. It can be substituted with either sage or coriander if you prefer.

1 Season the pork steaks on both sides with plenty of salt and freshly ground black pepper then place in a preheated non-stick pan.

2 Dry-fry on both sides for 5–6 minutes until lightly browned, then remove from the pan and place on a plate.

3 Add the onion and apples to the pan and cook gently until lightly coloured. Add the ginger and 2 tablespoons of stock. Sprinkle the flour over and cook out for 1 minute. Gradually stir in the remaining stock with the mushrooms and wine.

4 Return the pork to the pan and add the tarragon. Simmer gently for 15–20 minutes until the sauce has reduced and the pork is cooked through.

SERVES 4
PER SERVING:
298 KCAL/7G FAT
PREPARATION TIME:
20 MINUTES
COOKING TIME:
40 MINUTES

4 lean pork steaks
1 medium red onion, finely chopped
2 red eating apples, cored and chopped
1 × 2.5cm (1in) piece of fresh ginger, peeled and finely chopped
1 vegetable stock cube dissolved in 300ml (1/2 pint) water
1 tablespoon plain flour
225g (8oz) chestnut mushrooms, sliced
1 wine glass white wine
1 tablespoon chopped fresh tarragon

Pork Provençale

SERVES 4
PER SERVING:
315 KCAL/10.2G FAT
PREPARATION TIME:
10 MINUTES
COOKING TIME:
20 MINUTES

4 lean pork slices

1 medium red onion, finely
chopped

2 garlic cloves, crushed

1 small aubergine, finely diced

1 red pepper, seeded and finely
chopped

600ml (1 pint) tomato passata

2 teaspoons vegetable stock
powder

1 tablespoon chopped fresh
mixed herbs

salt and freshly ground black
pepper

*Quick and easy, these tender pork slices make a perfect tasty meal.
Cutting the vegetables into small dice allows them to cook much
quicker and also adds texture to the thick tomato sauce.*

1 Preheat a non-stick pan. Trim away any traces of fat from each
pork slice. Using a rolling pin, beat the pork into a thin slice,
then season generously with salt and freshly ground black
pepper. Seal the slices in a hot pan on both sides then remove
and keep warm.

2 Add the onion, garlic, aubergine and red pepper to the pan.
Cook quickly over a high heat to soften. Add the tomato
passata, stock powder and herbs, stir well then return the pork
to the pan. Cover and simmer for 5–6 minutes to allow the pork
to cook through.

3 Serve straight away with potatoes and a selection of fresh
vegetables.

Chinese spiced pork fillet

Lemon marmalade forms the base to a rich sticky sauce that is perfect for the finest cut of pork. This recipe also works well with duck breast, but do remember to remove the skin before cooking.

1 Preheat the oven to 200C, 400F, Gas Mark 6.
2 Trim away any fat from the pork and cut into 4 equal-sized pieces. Season well with salt and freshly ground black pepper and set aside.
3 Preheat a non-stick frying pan until hot. Carefully add the pork, turning quickly to seal all sides. Transfer to an ovenproof dish, place in the hot oven and continue cooking for 15–20 minutes.
4 Add the garlic to the pan and soften. Add the sherry and the remaining ingredients. Simmer gently until the pork is cooked.
5 Remove the pork from the oven and allow to rest for 4–5 minutes before slicing into medallions. Arrange on a serving plate and pour the sauce over.

SERVES 4
PER SERVING:
438 KCAL/10G FAT
PREPARATION TIME:
10 MINUTES
COOKING TIME:
35 MINUTES

1 kg (2lb) lean pork fillet
2 garlic cloves, finely chopped
50ml (2fl oz) dry sherry
2 tablespoons lemon
    marmalade
50ml (2fl oz) tomato passata
1 red chilli, finely chopped
½ teaspoon Chinese five spice
    powder
salt and freshly ground black
    pepper

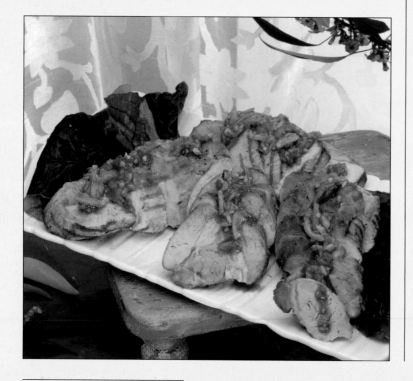

Balsamic pork chop with tangerine

SERVES 1
PER SERVING:
325 KCAL/8.2G FAT
PREPARATION TIME:
5 MINUTES
COOKING TIME:
12–15 MINUTES

1 lean pork chop or slice
1 orange
$\frac{1}{2}$ red pepper, seeded and finely
 diced
2 teaspoons good balsamic
 vinegar
2–3 basil leaves
1 tangerine, segmented
salt and freshly ground black
 pepper

This recipe requires a good balsamic vinegar, which will be thick and sweet, unlike cheaper types that are still quite sharp in flavour. The pork may be left in the marinade overnight to absorb all the flavours.

1 Remove all visible fat from the pork and place the pork in a shallow dish.
2 Using a zester, remove strands of peel from the orange and place on top of the pork. Cut the orange in half and squeeze the juice over the pork.
3 Scatter the red pepper over the pork and drizzle with balsamic vinegar.
4 Coarsely shred the basil leaves and add to the dish. Turn the pork over to coat both sides, cover and refrigerate for at least 1 hour.
5 Preheat a non-stick griddle pan until hot. Remove the pork from the marinade and season to taste.
6 Place the pork in the griddle pan and cook for 5–6 minutes on each side. Just before the end of cooking, add any marinade residue and the tangerine segments and heat through.

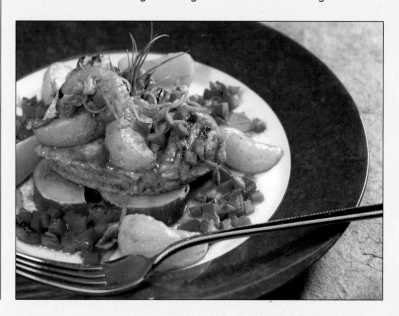

Grilled lamb steaks with cranberry and mint

Choose a lean cut of lamb such as fillet as opposed to fatty chops with very little lean meat. The meat can be marinated overnight in the refrigerator for added flavour.

1 Cut the lamb into steaks and place in a shallow dish. Sprinkle the rosemary and garlic over and season well with salt and freshly ground black pepper. Pour the orange juice over and leave to marinate for 30 minutes.
2 Remove the lamb from the marinade and place on a grill tray. Cook under a hot grill for 5–6 minutes each side.
3 Pour the marinade into a small saucepan, add the cranberries and cranberry sauce and heat gently.
4 Slake the cornflour with a little water and add to the sauce. Stir well until the sauce starts to thicken.
5 Arrange the lamb steaks on a serving dish, add the mint to the sauce and pour the sauce over. Serve with potatoes and a vegetable selection.

SERVES 4
PER SERVING:
285 KCAL/15G FAT
PREPARATION TIME:
10 MINUTES
COOKING TIME:
40 MINUTES

450g (1lb) lean lamb filet
2 garlic cloves, crushed
a few sprigs fresh rosemary
300ml (1/2 pint) fresh orange juice
50g (2oz) fresh cranberries
1 tablespoon cranberry sauce
1 tablespoon cornflour
2 tablespoons chopped fresh mint
salt and freshly ground black pepper

Griddled lamb's liver with tomato and bacon salsa

SERVES 4
PER SERVING:
405 KCAL/17G FAT
PREPARATION TIME:
25 MINUTES
COOKING TIME:
10 MINUTES

1kg (2lb) lamb's liver, sliced
2 garlic cloves, crushed
300ml (½ pint) semi-skimmed
  milk
salt and freshly ground black
  pepper
2 teaspoons oil (for lining the
  pan and then removed)

for the salsa
4 rashers lean back bacon
6 ripe tomatoes
4 sundried tomatoes, soaked in
  boiling water
1 lime
1 tablespoon chopped fresh
  chives
1 tablespoon balsamic vinegar
1 teaspoon clear honey
salt and freshly ground black
  pepper

Liver, bacon and tomatoes in a different style. The milk removes any bitterness from the liver as well as having a tenderising effect.

1 Place the liver in a shallow dish. Dot with the crushed garlic and pour the milk over. Allow to sit for 30 minutes while you make the salsa.

2 Make the salsa. Skin the tomatoes by plunging them into boiling water for 10 seconds. Remove and submerge in ice-cold water. Peel away the skin, then slice each tomato in half and remove the seeds, using a teaspoon.

3 Chop the tomato flesh and place in a bowl with the reconstituted sundried tomatoes. Using a zester, remove thin strips of zest from the lime and add to the bowl along with the juice. Stir in the chives, balsamic vinegar and honey, seasoning to taste.

4 Preheat a non-stick griddle pan, lightly greasing with a little oil and removing the excess with kitchen towel.

5 When the pan is very hot add the bacon and cook quickly for 4–5 minutes on each side until crisp. Remove from the pan and drain on kitchen paper before chopping into small pieces. Add to the salsa.

6 Wipe out the griddle pan, adding a little oil if necessary. Remove the liver from the milk and drain on kitchen paper. Add to the pan and cook quickly for 3–4 minutes on each side. If overcooked, the texture will become tough and rubbery.

7 Serve with the salsa.

Pot roast lamb with celery and peppers

A delicious lamb dish full of flavour. Choose a very lean piece of meat, as lamb is naturally high in fat. Other cuts of meat are equally suited such as silverside or topside of beef.

1 Preheat the oven to 180C, 350F, Gas Mark 4.
2 Using a small sharp knife, make incisions all over the lamb. Push slices of garlic and small sprigs of rosemary into the holes and season well with salt and pepper.
3 Preheat a non-stick frying pan until very hot. Add the lamb and quickly brown on all sides, then transfer the meat to an earthenware dish.
4 Add the onions, celery and peppers and cook until lightly coloured. Add 2–3 tablespoons of stock and sprinkle the flour over, cook briefly, then gradually mix in the remaining stock. If the pan is not sufficiently big enough to hold the total liquid transfer the mixture to the earthenware pot and add the remaining stock along with the tomato purée and lemon peel.
5 Cover the pot and place in the preheated oven for 2–2$\frac{1}{2}$ hours until tender.
6 Before serving, scoop off any fat from the top of the dish with a small ladle, then remove the meat from the sauce onto a serving plate. Adjust the consistency of the sauce by reducing in a saucepan over a high heat.
7 Serve with seasonal vegetables.

SERVES 4
PER SERVING:
353 KCAL/13.5G FAT
PREPARATION TIME:
15 MINUTES
COOKING TIME:
2 HOURS

1kg (2lb) leg of lamb, skin removed
2 garlic cloves, sliced
3–4 sprigs fresh rosemary
2 medium red onions, chopped
1 head celery, sliced
2 red peppers, seeded and sliced
1.2 litres (2 pints) meat stock
2 tablespoons plain flour
2 tablespoons tomato purée
2 pieces lemon peel
salt and freshly ground black pepper

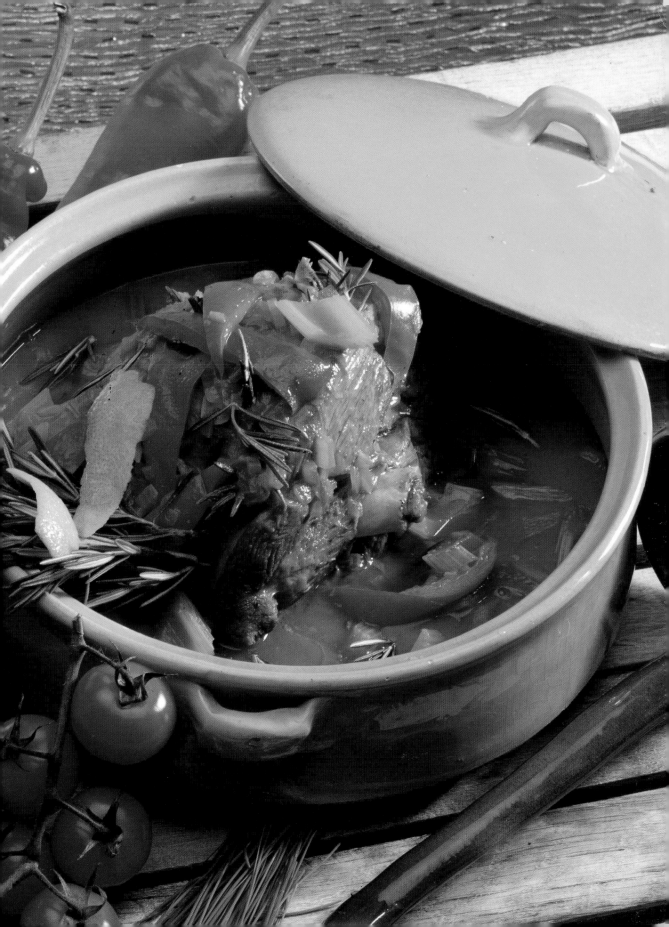

Kidneys in chilli tomato sauce

This chilli sauce is ideal to use hot or cold with grilled meat or fish. Always buy fresh kidneys for use straight away, as they are unsuitable even for short-term storage.

1 Preheat the grill to high.
2 Wash the kidneys well and slice open through the crescent side of the meat, not cutting right the way through but sufficient to be able to open out the kidney. Cut away any white core and splay open by inserting 2 cocktail sticks across each open kidney. Season well with salt and freshly ground black pepper.
3 In a non-stick frying pan dry fry the onion for 2–3 minutes until soft, add the garlic and pepper and cook for 2–3 minutes more.
4 Add the passata and chilli, bringing the sauce to a gentle simmer. Season to taste with salt and freshly ground black pepper.
5 Grill the kidneys for 5–8 minutes, depending on their size, turning frequently.
6 Place the kidneys on a serving dish and sprinkle with shredded basil leaves. Pour the sauce over and serve.

SERVES 4
PER SERVING:
156 KCAL/4.8G FAT
PREPARATION TIME:
20 MINUTES
COOKING TIME:
10 MINUTES

8 large kidneys
1 red onion, finely chopped
2 garlic cloves, crushed
1 red pepper, seeded and finely chopped
300ml ($\frac{1}{2}$ pint) tomato passata
1 red chilli, seeded and finely chopped
8–10 basil leaves
salt and freshly ground black pepper

Hattie's crunchy baked chicken

SERVES 4
PER SERVING:
106 KCAL/0.7G FAT
PREPARATION TIME:
10 MINUTES
COOKING TIME:
35 MINUTES

4 skinless chicken pieces
4 tablespoons spicy tomato
  chutney
4 handfuls cornflakes
salt and freshly ground black
  pepper
1 tablespoon chopped fresh
  coriander to garnish

This is a particular favourite with children. The crunchy coating tastes absolutely delicious – just as good as Southern Fried without the fat.

1 Preheat the oven to 200C, 400F, Gas Mark 6.
2 Place the chicken pieces in an ovenproof dish and season well with salt and freshly ground black pepper. Coat each piece of chicken thoroughly with the tomato chutney and place a thick layer on the top.
3 Crush the cornflakes by placing them in a plastic food bag and roll a rolling pin over or alternatively press between two large flat plates.
4 Roll the chicken pieces in the crushed cornflakes until totally coated, sprinkling any excess on the top.
5 Bake in the preheated oven for 30–35 minutes until thoroughly cooked. Check by inserting a knife into the thickest part of the meat. The juices should run clear when fully cooked. If in any doubt return to the oven for a further 10–15 minutes.
6 Just before serving, garnish with the coriander.

Jamaican jerk chicken

There are many variations of this spicy flavoursome chicken dish. This one uses Habanero or Scotch Bonnet chillies, some of the hottest chillies available. If your palate doesn't stretch to this heat scale, then substitute with the milder bullet variety or play safe with a little chilli sauce.

1 Prepare the chicken by removing all traces of fat and any white strands of sinew. Slash the flesh of each piece with a sharp knife several times and place in a non-metallic bowl. Season each piece well with salt and freshly ground black pepper.

2 Prepare the jerk seasoning by crushing the allspice berries in either a pestle and mortar or use the broad edge of a large chopping knife, pressing the berries against a solid chopping board. Place in a small glass bowl and add the red onion and garlic. Add the remaining ingredients except the coriander and mix well. Spread the mixture over the chicken, turning each piece to coat. Allow to marinate for 2–3 hours.

3 Cook the chicken either under a preheated hot grill or on a barbecue for approximately 20–25 minutes. It is very important to check the chicken is fully cooked through to the centre before serving. The juices should run clear when a knife is inserted into the thickest part of the chicken.

4 Just before serving, sprinkle with chopped coriander. Serve hot or cold with rice and a selection of salads.

SERVES 4
PER SERVING:
396 KCAL/5.8G FAT
PREPARATION TIME:
20 MINUTES
COOKING TIME:
25–30 MINUTES

8 pieces skinless chicken
  (drumstick, breast or thighs)
6–8 allspice berries
1 small red onion, finely
  chopped
2 garlic cloves, crushed
1 teaspoon finely chopped fresh
  ginger
½ teaspoon ground mace
1 Habanero or Scotch Bonnet
  chilli, finely chopped
2 tablespoons light soy sauce
zest and juice of 3 limes
2 tablespoons chopped fresh
  coriander
salt and freshly ground black
  pepper

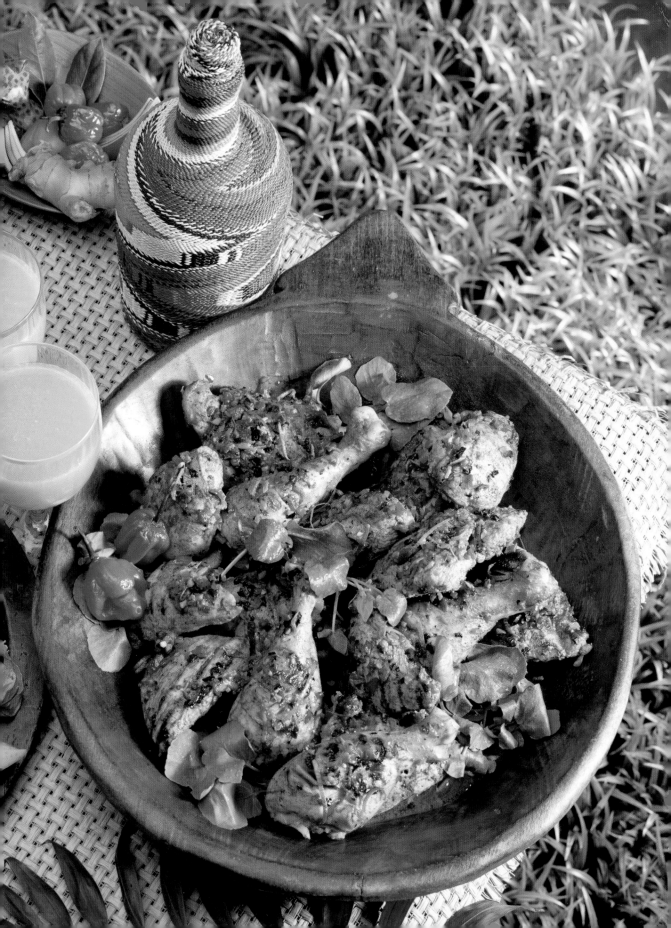

Preserved lemon chicken

Preserved lemons are a fundamental part of Moroccan cookery. The thin-skinned fruits are heavily salted and stored in a brine solution for a minimum of three weeks. The flavour is quite different to fresh lemons, as the salt draws out the bitter flavours of the lemon.

SERVES 4
PER SERVING:
265 KCAL/4.5G FAT
PREPARATION TIME:
15 MINUTES
COOKING TIME:
45 MINUTES

1 large onion, diced
450g (1lb) skinless chicken
    breasts, cut into pieces
2 garlic cloves, finely chopped
450ml (¾ pint) chicken stock
2 tablespoons plain flour
1 tablespoon chopped fresh
    sage
1 teaspoon fennel seeds
1 teaspoon ground cumin
6 cardamom pods, crushed
1 small red chilli, finely sliced
1 × 400g (14oz) can chopped
    tomatoes
1 preserved lemon, cut into
    quarters and core removed
salt and freshly ground black
    pepper

Preserving lemons

To preserve lemons, cut 2 large lemons into quarters. Place 50g (2oz) salt in a clean pint jar. Pack the lemons in and pour sufficient lemon juice over to cover. Seal the jar and shake to dissolve some of the salt. Keep in a cool place or refrigerator and shake the jar every day. It is ready to use at this point. It will keep indefinitely in a refrigerator.

---

1 In a non-stick pan dry-fry the onion until soft. Add the chicken and garlic and continue to cook until lightly coloured.

2 Add 2–3 tablespoons of stock to the pan, sprinkle the flour over and mix well, cooking the flour out for 1 minute. Gradually stir in the remaining stock.

3 Add the herbs and spices, tomatoes and preserved lemon. Cover and simmer gently for 20–25 minutes until the sauce thickens.

4 Season to taste and serve with either rice and sala, or potatoes and a variety of vegetables.

Hot coronation chicken

SERVES 4
PER SERVING:
312 KCAL/3.9G FAT
PREPARATION TIME:
15 MINUTES
COOKING TIME:
20 MINUTES

4 skinless chicken breasts, cut
   into chunks
2 medium onions, finely
   chopped
2 garlic cloves, crushed
1–2 tablespoons korma curry
   powder
1 vegetable stock cube,
   dissolved in 150ml (¼ pint)
   boiling water
1 tablespoon plain flour
300ml (½ pint) skimmed milk
1 tablespoon chopped fresh flat
   leaf parsley
2 tablespoons virtually fat free
   Normandy fromage frais
1 tablespoon spicy mango
   chutney
50g (2oz) seedless white grapes
salt and freshly ground black
   pepper

*A hot version of this very popular family dish. For variety
substitute the mango chutney with finely diced fresh mango and
serve with a jacket potato or rice.*

1 Season the chicken pieces with salt and pepper and dry-fry in a
   non-stick pan for 6–7 minutes until they start to colour.
   Remove from the pan and set aside.
2 Add the onions and garlic to the pan and cook gently until soft.
   Sprinkle the curry powder over and add 2 tablespoons of stock.
   Mix well, then add the flour and cook out for 1 minute.
   Gradually add the remaining stock and milk, stirring
   continuously to prevent any lumps forming.
3 Return the chicken to the pan and add the parsley. Simmer
   gently for 8–10 minutes to ensure the chicken is fully cooked.
   Remove from the heat, stir in the fromage frais, mango chutney
   and grapes and serve with boiled rice.

Thai chicken curry

Marinating the chicken overnight maximises the flavour of this very spicy curry. Once cooked, the finished curry can be stored chilled or frozen and reheated as required.

1 Make the paste by grinding all the ingredients in either a food processor or liquidiser.
2 Scrape the paste into a bowl then rinse out the food processor bowl with a little stock. Add the chicken pieces to the paste and mix well. Allow to marinate for a minimum of 1 hour or ideally overnight.
3 In a non-stick pan dry-fry the onion until soft, then add the chicken and cook for 5–6 minutes, stirring continuously. Add the remaining ingredients except the fresh coriander and simmer gently for 15–20 minutes until the sauce thickens and the chicken is fully cooked through.
4 Just before serving, stir in the fresh coriander.

SERVES 4
PER SERVING:
240 KCAL/3.3G FAT
MARINATING TIME:
1 HOUR
PREPARATION TIME:
25 MINUTES
COOKING TIME:
30 MINUTES

for the paste
3 garlic cloves, peeled
1 tablespoon ground coriander
$1/2$ teaspoon ground turmeric
$1/2$ teaspoon fenugreek seeds or ground fenugreek
2–3 small whole fresh chillies
seeds removed from 4 crushed cardamom pods

1 large red onion, finely chopped
4 large skinless chicken breasts, cut into pieces
2 tablespoons tomato purée
600ml (1 pint) chicken or vegetable stock
1 tablespoon tamarind paste or hot fruit chutney
4 kaffir lime leaves
2 tablespoons chopped fresh coriander

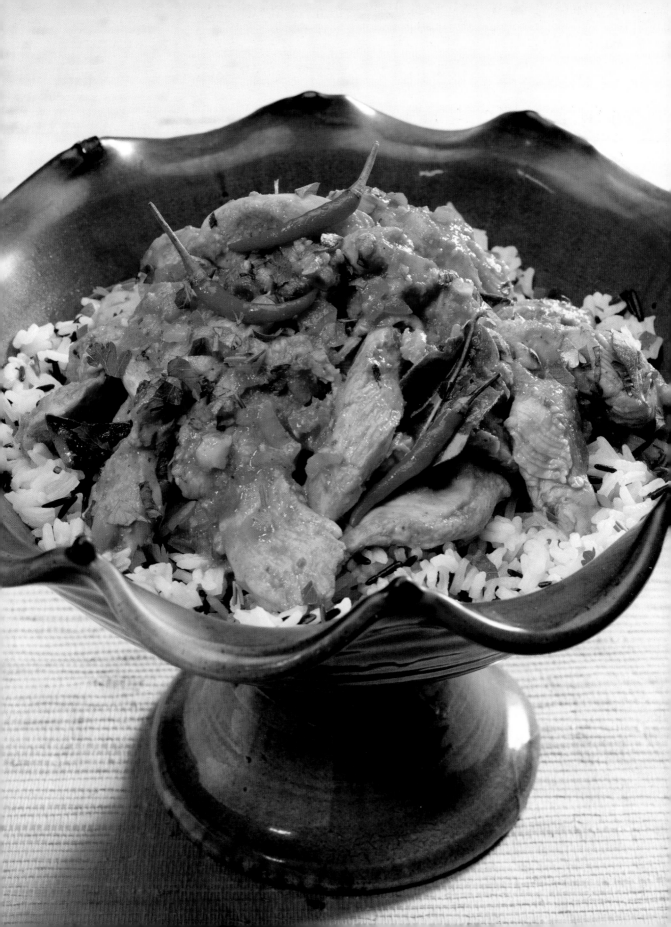

Chicken and coriander meat balls

These tasty chicken nuggets make ideal lunch box bites or picnic food. Serve hot tossed in a little tomato passata for a great pasta accompaniment.

1 Preheat the oven to 190C, 375F, Gas Mark 5.
2 Place all the ingredients in a large bowl and mix well. Mould the mixture into 16 small balls, each about the size of a golf ball, and place on a non-stick baking tray.
3 Bake in the oven for 20–25 minutes.
4 Serve hot with pasta and salad or cold with extra chutney.

SERVES 4
PER SERVING:
361KCAL/5.4G FAT
PREPARATION:
15 MINUTES
COOKING TIME:
20 MINUTES

1kg (2lb) lean minced chicken
1 small onion, finely chopped
1 garlic clove, crushed
2 teaspoons ground coriander
2 teaspoons ground cumin
1 tablespoon fruit chutney
2 tablespoons chopped fresh
   coriander
2 teaspoons vegetable bouillon
   stock powder
1 tablespoon tomato purée

Pancetta chicken with white wine

SERVES 4
PER SERVING:
321 KCAL/8.7G FAT
PREPARATION TIME:
20 MINUTES
COOKING TIME:
40 MINUTES

4 lean skinless chicken breasts
1 medium red onion, finely
  chopped
4 thin slices pancetta or smoked
  bacon
1 chicken stock cube dissolved in
  300ml (½ pint) water
1 tablespoon plain flour
225g (8oz) chestnut
  mushrooms, sliced
1 wine glass white wine
2 tablespoons chopped fresh
  mixed herbs

Pancetta is a lightly smoked cured Italian bacon. It adds good flavour to stocks and sauces. If unavailable, substitute smoked streaky bacon.

1 Season the chicken breasts on both sides with plenty of salt and freshly ground black pepper, then place in a preheated non-stick pan.
2 Dry-fry on both sides for 5–6 minutes until lightly browned, then remove from the pan and place on a plate.
3 Add the onion and pancetta to the pan and cook gently until lightly coloured. Add 2 tablespoons of stock. Sprinkle the flour over and cook out for 1 minute.
4 Gradually stir in the remaining stock with the mushrooms and wine.
5 Return the chicken to the pan and add the herbs. Simmer gently for 15–20 minutes until the sauce has reduced and the chicken has cooked through.

Hot pan smoked duck with orange salad

Pan smoking is a variation of barbecuing with the food being totally encased in the cooking smoke. The food is cooked in a smoker over wood chippings, adding flavour directly to the food (See page 184). Timing is essential as over-smoking can result in a dark film encasing the food, resulting in a strong bitter flavour.

1 Preheat the oven to 200C, 400F, Gas Mark 6.
2 Place the peppercorns in a pestle and mortar or grind between two flat plates.
3 Prepare the duck by removing the skin with a sharp knife. Season each breast well with salt and the peppercorns.
4 Prepare the smoker and place the duck pieces onto the wire rack. Cover the whole smoker with aluminium foil and stand the smoker over a low heat.
5 Smoke for 8–10 minutes, reducing the heat if the smoke smells strong.
6 Turn off the heat and allow the smoker to stand for 2–3 minutes before removing the foil. Transfer the duck to a baking tray and cover with the thyme sprigs, place in the preheated oven for 5–6 minutes to finish cooking.
7 Remove the duck from the oven and allow to rest for 5 minutes.
8 Segment the oranges by removing the outer skin and pith with a sharp knife. Cut in between the thin membrane, separating each orange segment.
9 Place the orange segments in a serving bowl and toss through the rocket leaves. Arrange on serving plates.
10 Drain away the meat juices from the duck into a small bowl and stir in the redcurrant jelly and the mint.
11 Slice the duck into pieces, add to the salad and drizzle with the dressing.

SERVES 4
PER SERVING:
195 KCAL/2.2G FAT
PREPARATION TIME:
5 MINUTES
COOKING TIME:
20 MINUTES

2 packs of 2 Gressingham skinless duck breasts (available from Sainsbury's)
salt
2 tablespoons mixed peppercorns
a few fresh sprigs thyme
4 large oranges
50g (2oz) fresh rocket leaves
1 tablespoon redcurrant jelly
a few fresh mint leaves, chopped

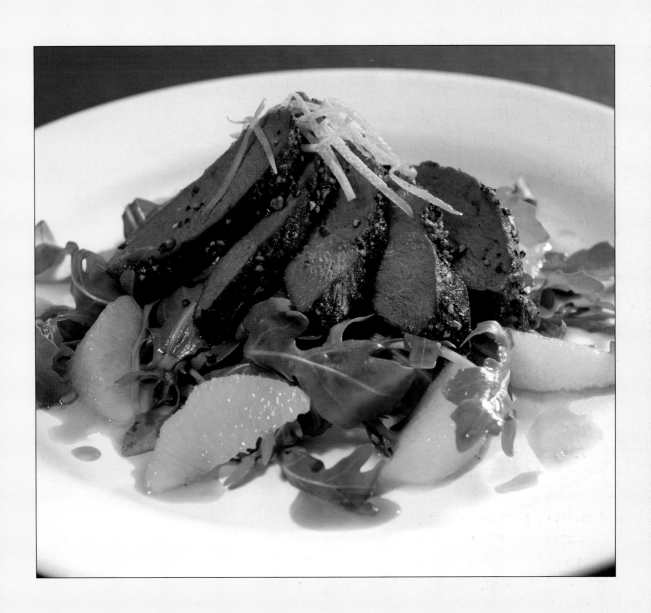

Fish and shellfish

Fresh fish is probably the easiest option on a low-fat diet. High in protein and naturally low in fat, bought prepared, it takes only minutes to cook in many versatile ways from steaming, grilling to baking and the barbecue.

Non-stick griddle pans are perfect for cooking firm, meaty fish steaks such as fresh tuna or swordfish. With the variety available, it makes sense to include fish more in our weekly menu planning.

Oily fish such as salmon and mackerel contains essential fatty acids, important for good health, and is therefore acceptable in moderation on a low-fat eating plan.

The key to maximising the flavour is to cook fish lightly, using fresh herbs and spices as a coating or sauce addition.

Lobster couscous salad

SERVES 4
PER SERVING:
270 KCAL/3.3G FAT
PREPARATION TIME:
20 MINUTES
COOKING TIME:
5 MINUTES

meat from 1 large cooked
    lobster
1 vegetable stock cube
    dissolved in 400ml (14fl oz)
    boiling water
1 teaspoon ground coriander
1 garlic clove, crushed
175g (6oz) couscous
1 tablespoon finely chopped
    chives
1 tablespoon chopped fresh
    coriander
4 tomatoes, skinned, seeded and
    diced
1/2 cucumber, peeled and diced
salt and freshly ground black
    pepper

for the dressing
150ml (1/4 pint) fresh apple juice
juice of 2 limes
1 tablespoon good quality white
    wine vinegar
1 teaspoon Dijon mustard
fresh coriander to garnish

Lobster turns a simple salad into a luxurious seafood delight. If you are unsure about how to prepare or cook lobster, then buy it freshly cooked and use straight away. For a vegetarian option cook the couscous in the same manner and top with a selection of oven roasted vegetables or dry-fried Quorn.

1 Cut the cooked lobster meat into bite-sized pieces.
2 In a large saucepan bring the stock to the boil, adding the ground coriander and garlic. Gradually pour in the couscous, stirring well. Cover with a lid, remove from the heat and allow to stand for 1 minute.
3 Remove the lid and, using 2 forks, fluff up the couscous grains. Add the herbs, tomato and cucumber and mix well, seasoning to taste.
4 Pile the couscous mixture into a serving dish and arrange the cooked lobster on top.
5 Combine the dressing ingredients and spoon over the lobster, sprinkle with fresh coriander and serve.

See photograph on page 110.

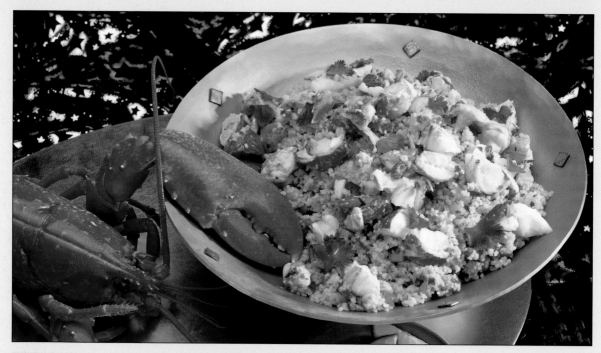

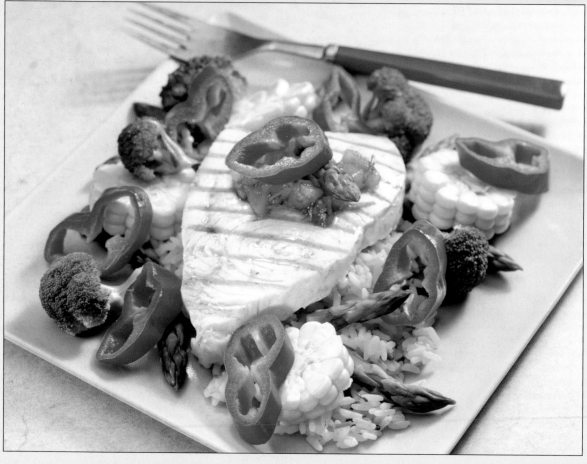

Griddled swordfish with tomato and lime salsa

SERVES 4
PER SERVING:
169 KCAL/5G FAT
PREPARATION TIME:
25 MINUTES
COOKING TIME:
10 MINUTES

4 fresh swordfish steaks

for the marinade
4 tablespoons light soy sauce
zest and juice of 2 limes
1 small red chilli, seeded and
    finely chopped
1 × 2.5cm (1in) piece fresh
    ginger, peeled and finely
    chopped
salt and freshly ground black
    pepper
2 teaspoons oil to line pan

for the salsa
6 ripe tomatoes
1 lime
1 tablespoon chopped fresh
    chives
1 tablespoon balsamic vinegar
salt and freshly ground black
    pepper

Top left: *Lobster couscous salad*

Left: *Griddled swordfish with
tomato and lime salsa*

1 Place the swordfish steaks in a shallow dish.
2 Combine all the marinade ingredients together in a small bowl and pour over the swordfish steaks. Leave to marinate for 20 minutes.
3 To make the salsa, skin the tomatoes by plunging them into boiling water for 10 seconds. Remove and submerge in ice-cold water. Peel away the skin, then slice each tomato in half and remove the seeds, using a teaspoon.
4 Chop the tomato flesh and place in a bowl. Using a zester, remove thin strips of zest from the lime and add to the bowl, along with the juice. Stir in the chives and balsamic vinegar. Season to taste.
5 Preheat a non-stick griddle pan, lightly greasing with a little oil and removing the excess with kitchen paper.
6 When the pan is very hot, carefully add the swordfish and season with salt and freshly ground black pepper. Cook it quickly for 4–5 minutes on each side. If overcooked the texture will become tough and rubbery.
7 Garnish with the salsa and serve hot.

Griddled monkfish with dill and lemon dressing

Monkfish is very dense and chunky in texture, making it ideal to griddle or barbecue. It needs very little cooking, although it does depend on the thickness of each tail. Because of its density, always make sure it is cooked through to the centre, but be careful not to overcook.

1 Prepare the monkfish by removing the thin outer skin and cut into chunky pieces. Season well with salt and freshly ground black pepper.
2 Preheat a non-stick griddle pan until hot, and cook the fish over a high heat for 2–3 minutes on each side. Remove from the pan and cover to keep warm.
3 Add the remaining ingredients except the fromage frais to the pan, stirring continuously to combine. Bring the dressing to a low simmer and return the sealed fish to the pan. Cover with a lid for 2–3 minutes until the fish is heated through.
4 Just before serving, stir in the fromage frais.

SERVES 4
PER SERVING:
184 KCAL/1.3G FAT
PREPARATION TIME:
20 MINUTES
COOKING TIME:
15 MINUTES

1 kg (2lb) monkfish tail fillets,
    boned and skinned
300ml (½ pint) apple juice
juice of 1 lemon
2 teaspoons Dijon mustard
2 teaspoons finely chopped dill
½ teaspoon ground fenugreek
1 teaspoon green peppercorns
    in brine
2 tablespoons virtually fat free
    Normandy fromage frais
salt and freshly ground black
    pepper

Bouillabaisse

SERVES 4
PER SERVING:
368 KCAL / 7.2G FAT
PREPARATION TIME:
20 MINUTES
COOKING TIME:
30 MINUTES

Probably the most famous fish stew, which has been adapted from a simple, peasant- style dish to a glamorous feast. It is traditionally served with either rouille, a rust orange garlic sauce, or aïoli (a garlic, olive oil and egg yolk sauce – see page 164 for a low-fat recipe). In this recipe you can use either small, whole, gutted fish or fish steaks cut from larger fish.

3 banana or French shallots,
   finely chopped
3 baby leeks, sliced
2 garlic cloves, finely chopped
good sprig of fresh thyme
$\frac{1}{2}$ teaspoon fennel seeds
2 pieces orange rind
1 small red chilli, finely chopped
good pinch of saffron
1 × 400g (14oz) can chopped
   tomatoes
1.2 litres (2 pints) fish stock
1kg (2lb) mixed fish (John Dory,
   bass, red snapper or mullet,
   monkfish, parrot fish)
salt and freshly ground black
   pepper

for the rouille
4 tablespoons fine breadcrumbs
1 tablespoon marinated red
   pimento peppers
1 garlic clove, crushed
2–3 tablespoons stock from the
   bouillabaisse

1 In a large shallow non-stick pan dry-fry the shallots, leeks and garlic until soft. Add the herbs and spices and continue cooking for 1–2 minutes. Pour the tomatoes and stock into the pan and bring to the boil.
2 Place the fish on top of the stock, cover with a lid and simmer gently for 15–20 minutes until the fish is cooked. Carefully lift the fish from the pan and place in warmed serving dishes.
3 Increase the heat and boil the sauce (reserve 2–3 tablespoons for the rouille) to reduce to a rich consistency. Pour the sauce over the fish.
4 To make the rouille, place all the ingredients into a food processor and blend until smooth. Season with salt and freshly ground black pepper.
5 Garnish the stew with the rouille and serve with aïoli and boiled new potatoes.

Seafood pie

As the fish is uncooked, it is essential the pie is cooked in a hot oven to get the heat through to the centre of the pie. If the pie starts to brown quickly, cover the top with foil and place lower in the oven to finish cooking.

N.B. The sauce may boil over the sides of the dish, so line the base of the oven with foil for easy cleaning.

1 Preheat the oven to 220C, 425 F, Gas Mark 7.
2 Boil the potatoes in a saucepan of salted water until well cooked. Drain and mash well until smooth, adding the fromage frais and seasoning well.
3 Remove the skin and bones from the smoked haddock and place in the bottom of an ovenproof dish. Add the prawns and mussels, if using.
4 Check the crab meat for pieces of shell or tendons and place on top.
5 Place the leeks and the fish stock in a medium-sized saucepan and cook for 1–2 minutes. Sprinkle the flour over and mix well. Cook out for 1 minute over a low heat, then add the white wine and mustard, beating well. Gradually add the skimmed milk, stirring continuously to prevent any lumps forming. Bring to the boil, allowing the sauce to thicken.
6 Pour the sauce over the fish and allow to cool, stirring in the chives. Cover with the potatoes, either using a fork or piping through a piping bag with a large star nozzle.
7 Bake in the oven for 30–40 minutes until golden.

SERVES 6
PER SERVING:
283 KCAL/3.5G FAT
PREPARATION TIME:
10 MINUTES
COOKING TIME:
40 MINUTES

675g (1 1/2lb) potatoes, peeled
2 tablespoons virtually fat free fromage frais
225g (8oz) smoked haddock
225g (8oz) peeled prawns
115g (4oz) smoked or cooked mussels (optional)
225g (8oz) fresh crab meat
2 baby leeks, finely chopped
150ml (1/4 pint) fish stock
1 tablespoon plain flour
1/2 wine glass white wine or sherry
2–3 teaspoons mild Dijon mustard
600ml (1 pint) skimmed milk
1 tablespoon freshly chopped chives
salt and freshly ground black pepper
chopped fresh parsley to garnish

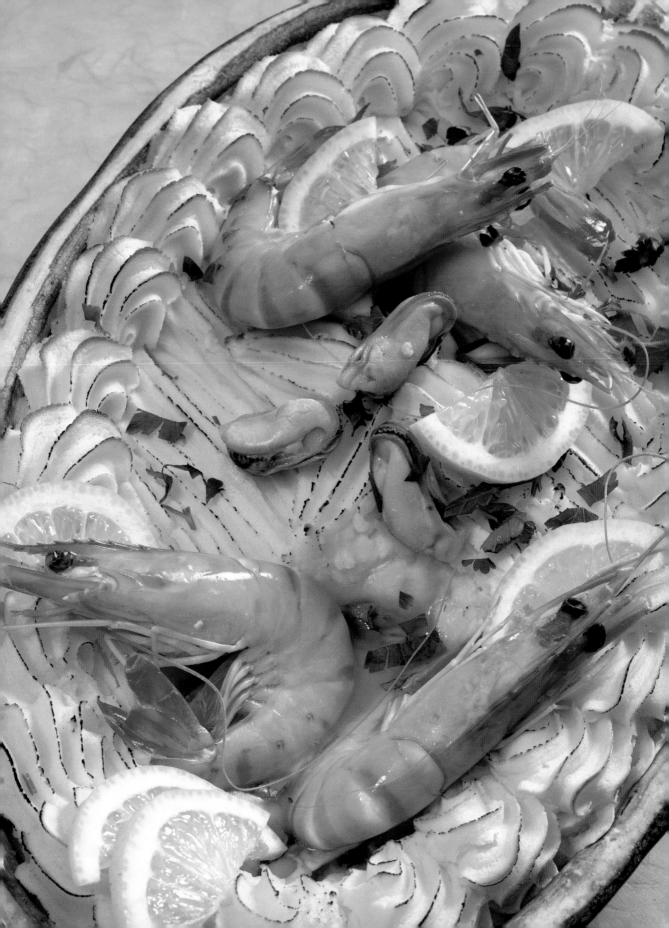

Vegetarian

We know that a good balance of nutritional meals is essential to our wellbeing. Eating some foods in excess, whether carbohydrates or protein-based foods such as meat, can have an adverse effect. With this in mind, many people now choose to incorporate vegetarian meals as part of their weekly plan.

It is essential to include foods from each of the four main food groups – proteins, milk and dairy products, cereals and grains, and fruit and vegetables.

Avoiding meat means you need to find alternative sources of protein in the form of beans and pulses. New plant-based products include TVP, tofu and Quorn, all of which can act as meat substitutes. Nuts stand alone since they are a high-fat commodity, so use sparingly.

Dairy products are essential for providing calcium. If wished, cow's milk may be substituted with soya milk and other vegetarian alternatives.

Look out for reduced-fat cheeses, particularly the mature type, which have a stronger flavour than the regular kind.

Carbohydrates such as bread, breakfast cereals, potatoes, pasta, rice and other grains should provide the bulk of food at every meal. Avoid serving these and vegetable accompaniments with additional fat. Use yogurt and low-fat cheese toppings. Serve pasta with tomato-based sauces, not cream-based, and use Parmesan shavings sparingly.

When preparing and cooking meals, you can reduce the fat by replacing oily marinades with fruit juices, soy sauce or diluted stock. Dry-frying and dry-roasting vegetables means that they cook successfully in their natural juices. Aubergine and mushrooms are a prime example, as these usually soak up oil or butter when fried.

Allow plenty of moisture in the form of well-flavoured herb stocks and tomato products such as passata or canned chopped tomatoes, which add volume as well as flavour.

If you choose not to eat fish, you may add a drop of oil to your cooking, one that is rich in essential fatty acids such as soya or rapeseed oil, but do use in moderation.

Quick vegetable korma

A quick and easy way to spice up vegetables. It is suitable for home freezing, so make up in a large batch and portion into small freezer containers. Once fully cooked, if liquidised it makes a great fresh curry sauce.

1 Preheat a non-stick pan, add the courgette, red pepper and mushrooms and dry-fry for 6–7 minutes until they start to colour.

2 Add the spring onions and garlic to the pan and cook gently until soft. Sprinkle the curry powder over and add 2 tablespoons of stock. Mix well, then add the flour and cook out for 1 minute.

3 Gradually add the remaining stock and the milk, stirring continuously to prevent any lumps from forming.

4 Add the parsley and simmer gently for 8–10 minutes. Remove from heat, stir in the fromage frais and serve with boiled rice.

SERVES 1
PER SERVING:
114 KCAL/1.5G FAT
PREPARATION TIME:
10 MINUTES
COOKING TIME:
15 MINUTES

1 courgette, sliced
1/2 red pepper, diced
2–3 chestnut mushrooms, sliced
4 spring onions, finely chopped
1 garlic clove, crushed
1–2 teaspoons korma curry powder
1 teaspoon vegetable bouillon stock powder, dissolved in 4 tablespoons boiling water
1 teaspoon plain flour
4 tablespoons skimmed milk
chopped fresh flat leaf parsley
1 tablespoon virtually fat free Normandy fromage frais
salt and freshly ground black pepper

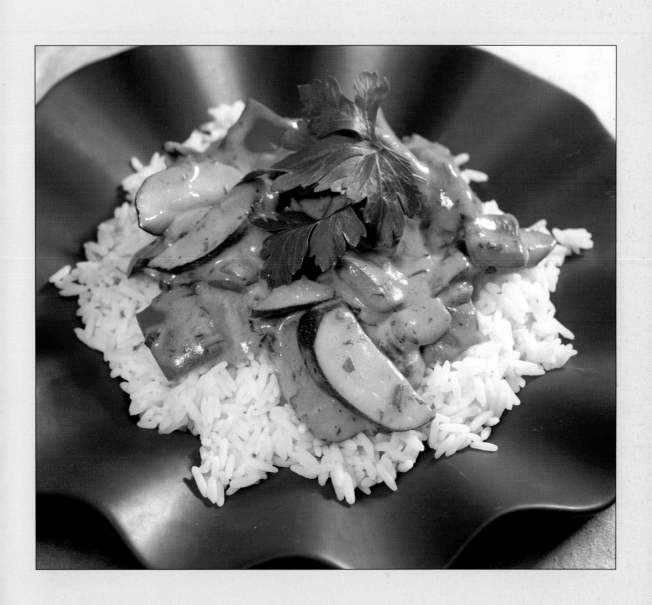

Navajo tortillas

These simple flat breads taste delicious eaten straight from the pan, but for ease cook them in advance and reheat for 4–5 minutes in a low oven. The mustard powder adds a golden colour as well as flavour.

1 Sieve all the dry ingredients into a large mixing bowl. Add the coriander and mix in.
2 Using a flat edged knife, make a well in the centre of the flour and slowly add sufficient milk, bringing the mixture together with the knife to form a soft dough.
3 Divide the dough into 8 equal balls. Using a rolling pin, roll out each ball onto a floured surface into a circle, getting the dough as thin as you can.
4 Stack the breads, dusting in between with flour.
5 Preheat a large non-stick frying or griddle pan until hot. Add a small amount of vegetable oil, then wipe out with a thick pad of kitchen paper.
6 Cook the tortillas in the hot pan for approximately 1 minute each side. Don't worry if the bread has black markings, as this will add flavour.
7 Stack the breads onto a warm plate and serve or reheat as required.

MAKES 8
PER TORTILLA:
209 KCAL/0.9G FAT
PREPARATION TIME:
5 MINUTES
COOKING TIME:
20 MINUTES

450g (1lb) soft white flour
1 teaspoon fine salt
2 teaspoons baking powder
2 teaspoons English mustard powder
2 tablespoons chopped fresh coriander
250–300ml (8–10fl oz) skimmed milk
a little vegetable oil

Pinto bean chilli burros

SERVES 4
PER SERVING:
242 KCAL/5G FAT
PREPARATION TIME:
15 MINUTES
COOKING TIME:
40 MINUTES

2 red onions, finely chopped

2 garlic cloves, crushed

2–3 fresh green chillies, seeded and chopped

2 thin courgettes, grated

1 × 400g (14oz) can pinto beans, drained and rinsed

1 × 400g (14oz) can chopped tomatoes

300ml (½ pint) tomato passata

2 teaspoons chopped fresh oregano

3 teaspoons vegetable bouillon stock powder

Pinto beans are beige in colour with brown speckles. They are native to Mexico but now mostly grown in the United States.

1 Preheat a non-stick frying pan. Dry-fry the onions and garlic for 1–2 minutes until soft. Add the chillies and courgettes and continue to cook for 2 minutes.

2 Stir in the remaining ingredients and bring to the boil. Reduce the heat and cover. Simmer gently for 20–25 minutes until the sauce thickens.

3 Serve as a filling for floured tortillas with shredded lettuce and chopped spring onion.

Cherry tomato and courgette tarte Tatin

A savoury version of the famous French apple tart. This vegetarian pie makes a great alternative to high-fat quiche and also works particularly well with roasted peppers.

1 Preheat the oven to 200C, 400F, Gas Mark 6.
2 Preheat a non-stick frying pan. Slice the tomatoes and arrange in the base of a 20cm (8in) ovenproof flan dish.
3 Dry-fry the courgettes quickly until coloured and add to the flan dish.
4 In a small saucepan heat the milk with the stock powder, mustard and garlic. Slake the cornflour with a little milk and add to the saucepan, whisking well. Simmer until the sauce thickens, stir in the herbs and cheese and pour onto the tomatoes and courgettes.
4 Beat together the egg and milk.
5 When the sauce is cool, place a sheet of pastry on top of the sauce, brush with beaten egg and milk, then add another layer of pastry. Continue until all the pastry is used up.
6 Brush the top and place in the oven for 20–25 minutes.
7 Allow to cool for 5 minutes, then turn out onto a tray or large serving plate.

SERVES 4
PER SERVING:
265 KCAL / 5.9G FAT
PREPARATION TIME:
10 MINUTES
COOKING TIME:
35 MINUTES

12 large cherry tomatoes
3 small courgettes, sliced
300ml (½ pint) skimmed milk
1 teaspoon vegetable bouillon stock powder
1 tablespoon Dijon mustard
1 garlic clove, crushed
1 tablespoon cornflour
2 tablespoons chopped fresh mixed herbs
50g (2oz) low-fat Cheddar cheese
1 egg
2 tablespoons skimmed milk
8 sheets filo pastry

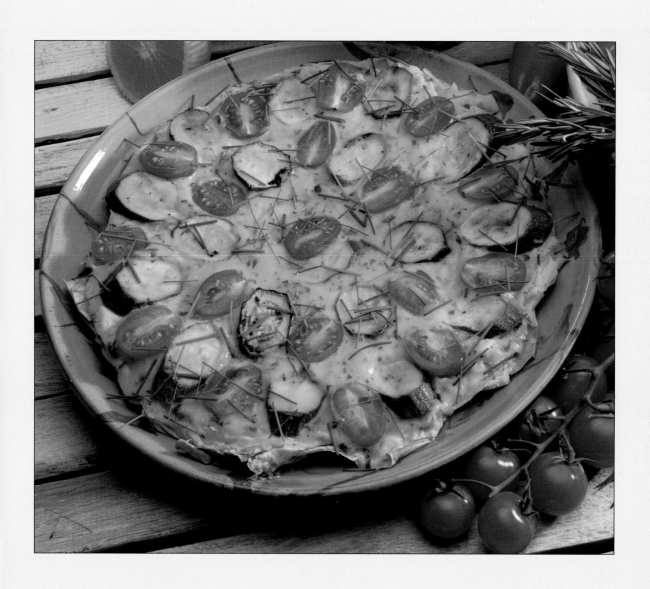

Potato and spinach soufflé

The secret of a good soufflé is to make sure the mixture is well beaten before adding the egg whites, then gently fold in the whites, retaining as much air as possible. The soufflé will start to deflate as soon as it leaves the oven, so serve straight away.

1 Preheat the oven to 180C, 350F, Gas Mark 4.
2 Place the potatoes in large bowl and, using a potato masher, mash well to remove any lumps. Beat in the fromage frais, garlic, egg yolks and spinach. Season well with salt and black pepper and a little nutmeg if desired. Add the grated cheese, reserving a pinch for later, and mix well.
3 In a clean bowl, whisk the egg whites until stiff. Fold into the mixture until fully combined and pour into a lightly greased 18cm (7in) soufflé dish.
4 Sprinkle the reserved cheese over the top and bake in the oven for 30–35 minutes until well risen and golden brown. Serve straight away with salad or vegetables.

SERVES 4
PER SERVING:
147 KCAL/6.4G FAT
PREPARATION TIME:
15 MINUTES
COOKING TIME:
55 MINUTES

225g (8oz) cooked potatoes
1 tablespoon virtually fat free
    fromage frais
1 garlic clove, crushed
3 eggs, separated
225g (8oz) fresh leaf spinach,
    stalked and finely shredded
grated fresh nutmeg (optional)
25g (1oz) grated low-fat
    Cheddar cheese
salt and freshly ground black
    pepper

Ribbon vegetable stir-fry

SERVES 4

PER SERVING:

186 KCAL/2.9G FAT

PREPARATION TIME:

20 MINUTES

COOKING TIME:

10 MINUTES

2 carrots

2 small parsnips

2 small courgettes

1 red pepper, seeded and finely
sliced

4 baby leeks, sliced

2 teaspoons finely chopped
fresh ginger

1 tablespoon light soy sauce

2 tablespoons chopped fresh
chives

115g (4oz) fine noodles

1 vegetable stock cube

zest and juice of 1 lime

1 medium red onion, finely
sliced

2 garlic cloves, crushed

*This large quantity of thinly sliced vegetables soon cooks down
when tossed in a hot pan. However, I find they are best cooked in
batches to ensure they cook evenly. Reheat in a moderate oven,
then toss with the hot noodles.*

1   Prepare the vegetables by peeling if required, then, using a
    vegetable peeler, take thin strips from the length of the carrots,
    parsnips and courgettes. Place in a bowl with the other
    vegetables, add the ginger, soy sauce and half of the chives.
    Mix well.

2   Cook the noodles in a pan of water containing a vegetable
    stock cube. Drain and toss with the lime zest and juice.

3   Heat a non-stick wok or frying pan, add the onion and garlic
    and cook until soft.

4   Add the vegetables and cook quickly over a high heat until they
    are just cooked.

5   Add the noodles and mix together well.

6   Serve in warmed bowls and sprinkle with the remaining
    chopped chives.

Spiced creamy vegetables with coconut milk

The perfect light summer curry. Coconut adds sweetness to the creamy sauce as well as a thickening agent. Serve with a sweet mango chutney and cucumber salad.

1 In a small saucepan boil together the coconut, carrots and milk for 10 minutes, then set aside.
2 In a preheated non-stick pan dry-fry the onions and garlic until soft, add the thyme and spices and continue cooking for a further 2 minutes.
3 Add 3 tablespoons of stock, then stir in the flour, cooking it out over a low heat.
4 Gradually stir in the remaining stock and the hot milk mixture.
5 Add the remaining vegetables and simmer gently until the vegetables are tender.

SERVES 4
PER SERVING:
253 KCAL/10.9G FAT
PREPARATION TIME:
20 MINUTES
COOKING TIME:
35 MINUTES

50g (2oz) desiccated coconut
450g (1lb) young tender carrots, scraped
600ml (1 pint) skimmed milk
2 medium onions, finely chopped
2 garlic cloves, crushed
2 teaspoons fresh thyme, chopped
$\frac{1}{2}$ teaspoon allspice
2 teaspoons ground cumin
1 teaspoon ground turmeric
1 tablespoon chopped fresh ginger
2 red chillies, finely chopped
150ml ($\frac{1}{4}$ pint) strong vegetable stock
1 tablespoon plain flour
4 baby leeks, finely chopped
225g (8oz) baby asparagus
115g (4oz) baby broad beans, shelled
115g (4oz) green beans

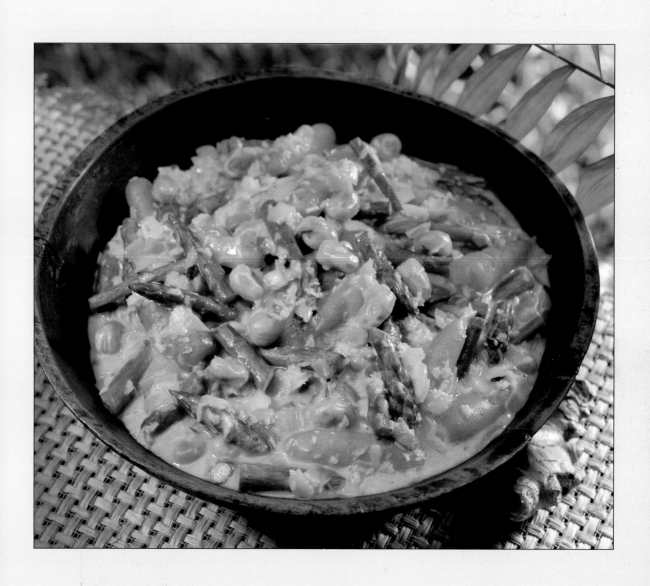

Wet polenta with Gorgonzola sauce

Polenta is made from ground corn or maize. It offers an alternative to potatoes or pasta. Although virtually all cheese is high in fat, the stronger-flavoured types can be used in small quantities when coupled with a low-fat base such as polenta or a jacket potato.

1 Weigh the polenta flour into a large jug so that it can be poured easily.
2 In a large saucepan bring the stock to the boil. Add the herbs and half the garlic, then slowly pour in the polenta flour in a continuous stream, stirring with a whisk to prevent lumps forming. Change the whisk for a wooden spoon and beat well until smooth. Reduce the heat to a gentle simmer and cook for 40–45 minutes, stirring occasionally.
3 Make the sauce by dry-frying the shallots and remaining garlic in a non-stick pan. Add the sherry and 2 tablespoons milk. Sprinkle the flour over and cook out for 1 minute, adding a little extra milk if it seems dry. Gradually mix in the remaining milk, add the sage and simmer to allow the sauce to thicken.
4 Just before serving, beat the fromage frais into the polenta, season well with salt and black pepper, add the crumbled Gorgonzola to the sauce and check the seasoning.
5 Arrange the polenta on a serving plate, pour the sauce over, then sprinkle with chopped coriander.

SERVES 4
PER SERVING:
340 KCAL/5G FAT
PREPARATION TIME:
10 MINUTES
COOKING TIME:
45 MINUTES

225g (8oz) Bramata polenta flour
1.2 litres (2 pints) vegetable stock
1 tablespoon chopped fresh mixed herbs
3 garlic cloves, crushed
2 long shallots, finely chopped
1 tablespoon dry sherry
600ml (1 pint) semi-skimmed milk
1 heaped tablespoon plain flour
1 teaspoon chopped fresh sage
2 tablespoons virtually fat free fromage frais
50g (2oz) Gorgonzola cheese, crumbled
salt and freshly ground black pepper
1 tablespoon chopped fresh coriander to garnish

Roasted vegetable curry

SERVES 4
PER SERVING:
148 KCAL/5.6G FAT
PREPARATION TIME:
15 MINUTES
COOKING TIME:
45 MINUTES

1 small aubergine, diced

2 red peppers, seeded and diced

2 yellow peppers, seeded and diced

1 red onion, chopped

2 courgettes, sliced

12 cherry tomatoes

2 garlic cloves, crushed

1 tablespoon mild curry powder

2 tablespoons light soy sauce

600ml (1 pint) tomato passata

seeds from 8 crushed cardamom pods

salt and freshly ground black pepper

1 tablespoon chopped fresh coriander

Try this recipe with many different combinations of vegetables. For a creamy sauce stir in 2 tablespoons of virtually fat free fromage frais just before serving.

1 Preheat the oven to 200C, 400F, Gas Mark 6.

2 Place all the vegetables in a non-stick roasting tray and season well with salt and black pepper. Dot with crushed garlic and sprinkle the curry powder over. Drizzle with the soy sauce and place in the top of the preheated oven. Roast for 20–25 minutes until the vegetables start to soften.

3 In a large saucepan heat the passata with the cardamom and add the cooked vegetables. Simmer over a low heat for 15 minutes to allow the sauce to thicken.

4 Check the seasoning, add the fresh coriander and serve.

French bread margarita

An express low-fat pizza for when you have little time to spare. However, do make sure you spread the mixture right up to the edges of the bread, as they may burn slightly when the baguette is returned to the grill.

1 Preheat the grill to high.
2 Lightly toast the bread on both sides, then using the cut side of the garlic rub the top of the toasted bread, pressing the centre down.
3 Empty the tomatoes into a small bowl. Mix in the basil leaves and season well with salt and black pepper.
4 Spread the mixture onto both pieces of bread, making sure it goes right up to the outside edges, and top with the sliced tomato.
5 In a small bowl mix together the salad dressing and cheese and spread on the top. Return to the grill until brown and bubbling.
6 Serve straight away with a mixed salad.

SERVES 1
PER SERVING:
214 KCAL/4G FAT
PREPARATION TIME:
5 MINUTES
COOKING TIME:
15 MINUTES

1 small French baguette, split in half lengthways
1 garlic clove, peeled and cut in half
1 × 115g (4oz) can chopped tomatoes
4–5 fresh basil leaves
1 tablespoon low-fat salad dressing
1 tablespoon grated low-fat Cheddar cheese
8 cherry tomatoes, sliced
salt and freshly ground black pepper

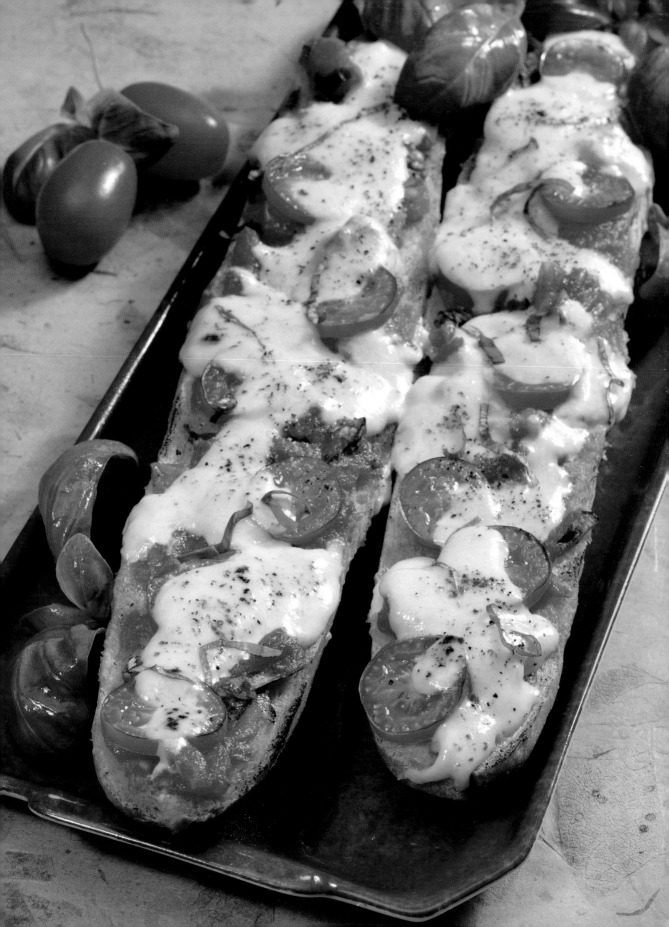

Lentil and roast vegetable loaf

Although the loaf can be served straight from the oven, it is best if allowed to cool and set completely and then reheated as required either as a whole or sliced.

1 Preheat the oven to 200C, 400F, Gas Mark 6.
2 Place the prepared vegetables into a roasting tin, season well with salt and black pepper and bake at the top of the oven for 25–30 minutes until lightly roasted.
3 In a saucepan bring to the boil the lentils, tomatoes, stock, garlic and thyme. Simmer for 15 minutes to soften the lentils and allow them to absorb the liquid. Mix the lentil mixture with the vegetables in a mixing bowl, adding the beaten egg.
4 Pour the mixture into a lightly greased 1kg (2lb) loaf tin and stand in a baking tray containing 2.5cm (1in) water. Bake in the middle of the oven for 40 minutes until risen and set. Allow to cool slightly before serving.
5 Just before serving, sprinkle with fresh basil.

SERVES 4
PER SERVING:
258 KCAL / 4.8G FAT
PREPARATION TIME:
25 MINUTES
COOKING TIME:
40 MINUTES

2 medium onions, finely chopped
2 courgettes, diced
1 small aubergine, diced
1 large red pepper, seeded and diced
175g (6oz) red lentils
1 × 400g (14oz) can chopped tomatoes
150ml (¼ pint) vegetable stock
2 garlic cloves, crushed
2 teaspoons chopped fresh thyme
2 eggs, beaten
salt and freshly ground black pepper
fresh basil to garnish

Spanish omelette

SERVES 1
PER SERVING:
238 KCAL/13.5G FAT
PREPARATION TIME:
10 MINUTES
COOKING TIME:
10 MINUTES

$\frac{1}{2}$ red onion, finely sliced
$\frac{1}{2}$ red pepper seeded and diced
1 garlic clove, crushed
1 tomato, skinned, seeded and
  finely diced
2 eggs, beaten and seasoned
  with salt and freshly ground
  black pepper

As the vegetables will release liquid when they are dry-fried, there is no need to add any milk to the egg mixture, although a teaspoon or two could be added if desired.

1 Preheat a non-stick frying pan. Dry-fry the onion, pepper and garlic for 3–4 minutes until soft.
2 Add the beaten egg and cook gently, using a wooden spatula to bring the set mixture from around the outside of the pan into the centre.
3 When the omelette is almost set, add the chopped tomato and turn the omelette over, either whole or split down the centre to make it easier.

Pasta and rice

There are many different types of pasta available with varying ingredients. Some use higher quantities of egg yolk than others, so check the labels carefully when buying dried pasta, as this can increase the calorie and fat content. Shapes and styles vary from fine noodles to large shapes suitable for filling. All require cooking in a large quantity of boiling water. Adding a vegetable or herb stock cube to the water does away with the need to use olive oil, which is usually added. The same applies to cooking rice, as the stock cube adds flavour to the cooking liquor. Always rinse rice well under cold running water before cooking to remove some of the starches. This will help keep the rice fluffy and loose once cooked.

Generally pasta and rice are low in fat; it is just the additions that bump up the fat grams, so choose tomato-based sauces and add chopped herbs such as basil or coriander to your stock boiled rice.

Allow 25g (1oz) dry weight pasta per person when serving as a starter and 50g (2oz) dry weight per person when serving as a main course.

Mushroom stir-fry with lemon noodles

SERVES 4
PER SERVING:
148 KCAL/2.7G FAT
PREPARATION TIME:
10 MINUTES
COOKING TIME:
10 MINUTES

115g (4oz) fine noodles

1 vegetable stock cube

zest and juice of 1 lemon

1 medium red onion, finely
    sliced

2 garlic cloves, crushed

450g (1lb) assorted mushrooms,
    sliced

2 teaspoons fresh ginger, peeled
    and finely chopped

1 tablespoon light soy sauce

chopped fresh chives to garnish

1 Cook the noodles in a pan of water containing a vegetable
   stock cube. Drain and toss with the lemon zest and juice.
2 Heat a non-stick wok or frying pan, add the onion and garlic,
   cooking until soft. Add the mushrooms, ginger and soy sauce.
   Cook quickly over a high heat until the mushrooms are just
   cooked.
3 Add the noodles and mix well together.
4 Serve in warmed bowls and sprinkle with chopped chives.

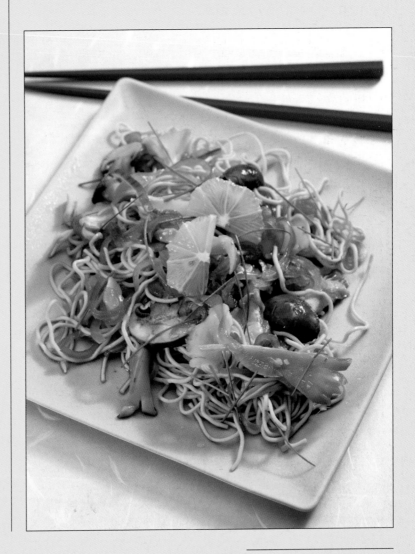

Three pepper rice

Adding just a few spices to rice really makes quite a difference. Kaffir lime leaves add a unique flavour. If you have difficulty in obtaining them, try fresh bay leaves as a substitute.

1 In a preheated non-stick pan dry-fry the onion and garlic until soft. Add the coriander seed and continue to cook for 3–4 minutes.

2 Add the saffron, rice and stir in the stock. Bring to the boil, adding the Kaffir lime leaves. Reduce the heat and cover with a lid.

3 Simmer gently for 20 minutes until all the stock has been absorbed, adding a little more stock if the mixture appears a little dry.

4 Once the rice is fully cooked add the diced peppers and stir well. Taste, adjusting the seasoning as required, and transfer to a warmed serving dish. Garnish with lemon and lime.

SERVES 4
PER SERVING:
199 KCAL/2G FAT
PREPARATION TIME:
15 MINUTES
COOKING TIME:
30 MINUTES

1 medium onion, finely chopped
1 garlic clove, crushed
1 teaspoon crushed coriander seed
good pinch of saffron
175g (6oz) basmati rice
450ml (¾ pint) vegetable stock
2 Kaffir lime leaves (optional)
1 red, 1 green, 1 yellow pepper, seeded and diced
salt and freshly ground black pepper
lemon and lime to garnish

Szechuan noodles

SERVES 4
PER SERVING:
161 KCAL／1G FAT
PREPARATION TIME:
10 MINUTES
COOKING TIME:
10 MINUTES

115g (4oz) dried noodles

2 vegetable stock cubes

4 spring onions, finely sliced

1 green pepper, seeded and
   finely sliced

1 celery stick, finely chopped

1 × 2.5cm (1in) piece ginger,
   peeled and finely chopped

115g (4oz) peeled prawns,
   chopped

1 small red chilli, sliced

2 tablespoons brandy

1 tablespoon soy sauce

1 tablespoon tomato purée

4 tablespoons vegetable stock

This is a great dish for using up odds and ends of vegetables, so vary according to your taste. If you wish, you can replace the prawns with finely chopped ham or extra vegetables.

1 Cook the noodles in boiling water, adding the stock cubes for extra flavour.
2 Preheat a non-stick wok or frying pan. Dry-fry the onions, pepper, celery and ginger together until lightly coloured.
3 Add the prawns and chilli and continue cooking for 2–3 minutes. Stir in the remaining ingredients, taking the vegetable stock from the noodle pan.
4 Drain the noodles and add to the vegetables. Mix well and serve.

Chicken spaghetti

1 Cook the spaghetti in a large pan of boiling water with a stock cube added for extra flavour.
2 In a non-stick pan dry-fry the onions and garlic until soft. Add the chicken, cooking until it completely changes colour. Add 2 tablespoons of stock and stir in the flour.
3 Cook out the flour for 1 minute, then gradually stir in the passata and herbs, seasoning with salt and black pepper. Reduce the heat and simmer for 2–3 minutes until the sauce thickens.
4 Drain the spaghetti and pour into a warmed serving dish. Spoon the sauce on top and garnish with chopped chives or rocket.

SERVES 4
PER SERVING:
312 KCAL/5.7G FAT
PREPARATION TIME:
10 MINUTES
COOKING TIME:
20 MINUTES

225g (8oz) [dry weight] spaghetti
1 vegetable stock cube
6 spring onions, finely chopped
1 garlic clove, crushed
115g (4oz) minced chicken
150ml ($\frac{1}{4}$ pint) vegetable stock
1 tablespoon plain flour
300ml ($\frac{1}{2}$ pint) tomato passata
1 tablespoon chopped fresh mixed herbs
salt and freshly ground black pepper
a few chopped fresh chives or some fresh rocket to garnish

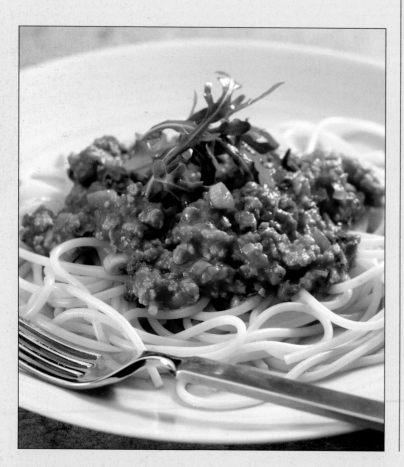

Pasta Sombrero

SERVES 4
PER SERVING:
296 KCAL/7.5G FAT
PREPARATION TIME:
10 MINUTES
COOKING TIME:
25 MINUTES

225g (8oz) pasta shapes

1 vegetable stock cube

1 small red onion, finely chopped

2 smoked garlic cloves, crushed

$\frac{1}{4}$ teaspoon fennel seeds

1 red and 1 green pepper, finely
   diced

pinch of sweet paprika

1 small red chilli, finely chopped

450g (16oz) tomato passata

1 teaspoon vegetable bouillon
   stock

a few anchovy fillets to garnish
   (optional)

The taste of Spain filters through this peppery pasta dish. Try to get the Sombrero pasta shapes or alternatively use other large shapes. You can buy smoked garlic.

1 Cook the pasta in a large saucepan of boiling water containing the stock cube.

2 In a preheated non-stick pan dry-fry the onion until soft. Add the garlic and fennel seeds and continue cooking for 2–3 minutes.

3 Add the remaining ingredients and simmer gently for 5–6 minutes.

4 Drain the pasta thoroughly and arrange on warmed serving plates. Carefully fill the pasta with the sauce.

5 Garnish with thinly sliced anchovy fillets if desired.

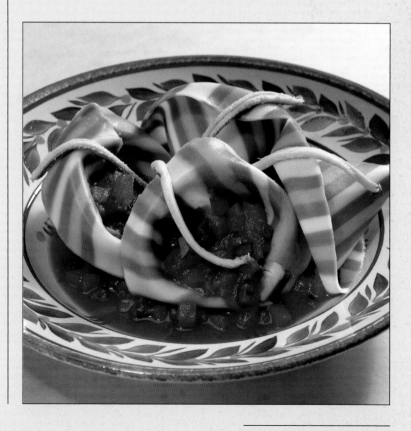

Leek and sundried tomato risotto

Sundried tomatoes can be found in most food shops. Avoid the type in oil, but if there is no alternative, then rinse well with hot water to remove as much oil as possible.

1 In a non-stick pan, dry-fry the leeks and garlic until soft.
2 Add the rice and tomatoes, then gradually stir in the stock and wine, allowing the rice to absorb it before adding more – this will take between 15 and 20 minutes.
3 Once all the liquid has been added stir in the vegetables and cover, allowing the vegetables to cook in the steam.
4 Fold in the fromage frais and remove from heat. Season with salt and black pepper. Serve hot with a little Parmesan cheese.

SERVES 4
PER SERVING:
305 KCAL/5.5G FAT
PREPARATION TIME:
10 MINUTES
COOKING TIME:
25 MINUTES

8 baby leeks, finely chopped
2 garlic cloves, crushed
225g (8oz) [dry weight] Arborio risotto rice
12 sundried tomatoes (not in oil), chopped
600ml (1 pint) vegetable stock
115g (4oz) baby asparagus
115g (4oz) frozen peas
2 tablespoons virtually fat free Normandy fromage frais
salt and freshly ground black pepper
3 tablespoons grated Parmesan cheese to serve

Smoked trout pasta bake

SERVES 4
PER SERVING:
310 KCAL/2.1G FAT
PREPARATION TIME:
10 MINUTES
COOKING TIME:
40 MINUTES

225g (8oz) pasta shapes

1 medium onion, finely chopped

2 garlic cloves, crushed

150ml ($\frac{1}{4}$ pint) vegetable stock

2 tablespoons plain flour

$\frac{1}{2}$ wine glass white wine

300ml ($\frac{1}{2}$ pint) skimmed milk

2 teaspoons Dijon mustard

1 tablespoon chopped fresh
chives

225g (8oz) smoked trout fillets,
flaked

3 tablespoons low-fat fromage
frais

salt and freshly ground black
pepper

A creamy pasta dish with wine and smoked trout to add contrasting flavours. For a vegetarian option replace the trout with roasted peppers and top with 50g (2oz) low-fat Cheddar.

1 Preheat the oven to 200C, 400F, Gas Mark 6.
2 Cook the pasta in boiling salted water until *al dente* (just tender), drain and rinse with cold water and place into a large bowl.
3 In a non-stick frying pan dry-fry the onion and garlic until soft. Add 2 tablespoons of stock, sprinkle the flour over, stir well and cook out for 1 minute before adding the remaining stock.
4 Gradually stir in the wine, milk and mustard and simmer gently for 2–3 minutes to allow the sauce to thicken.
5 Mix the sauce into the pasta, along with the chives, trout and fromage frais and season with salt and black pepper.
6 Pour into an ovenproof dish and bake in the preheated oven for 15–20 minutes until hot.

Aubergine and spinach pasta bake

This combination of vegetables works really well with the spicy tomato sauce. It can be made in advance and freezes very well.

1 Preheat the oven to 190C, 375F, Gas Mark 5.
2 Cook the pasta in boiling salted water with a vegetable stock cube. Drain well then stir in the shredded spinach.
3 Meanwhile, in a non-stick frying pan, dry-fry the onion for 2–3 minutes until soft, add the aubergine, garlic and red pepper and cook for a further 6–8 minutes until the aubergine starts to colour.
4 Add the tomatoes, chilli and remaining stock cube, bringing the sauce to a gentle simmer. Season to taste with salt and black pepper.
5 Pour the pasta into a large serving dish, cover with the sauce and sprinkle with the shredded basil leaves and grated cheese.
6 Bake in the preheated oven for 15–20 minutes until golden brown.
7 Serve with a mixed salad or fresh vegetables.

SERVES 4
PER SERVING:
300 KCAL/6.6G FAT
PREPARATION TIME:
10 MINUTES
COOKING TIME:
30 MINUTES

175g (6oz) [dry weight] shell or rigatoni-style pasta
2 vegetable stock cubes
225g (8oz) young spinach leaves, shredded
1 red onion, finely chopped
1 aubergine, diced
2 garlic cloves, crushed
1 red pepper, seeded and finely chopped
1 × 400g (14oz) can chopped tomatoes
1 red chilli, seeded and finely chopped
8–10 basil leaves, shredded
115g (4oz) low-fat Cheddar cheese, grated
salt and freshly ground black pepper

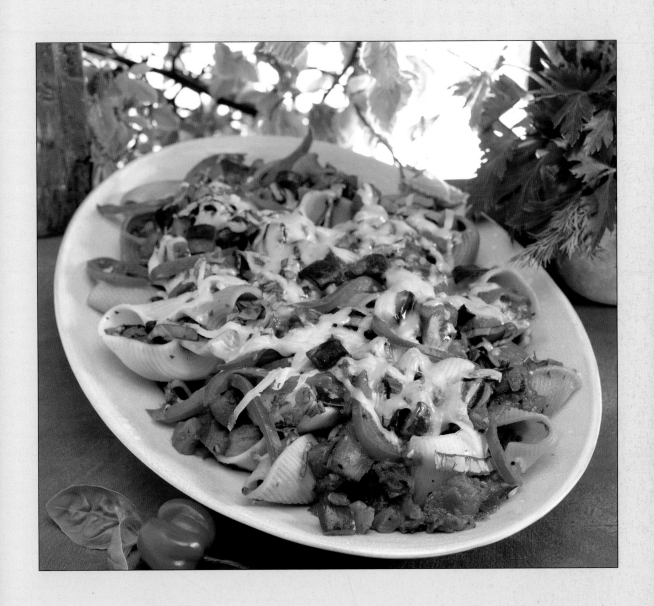

Puddings

In this chapter you'll find a great selection of traditional and some more unusual sweet offerings, both hot and cold, that keep fat to a minimum. All are easy to prepare – some need to be prepared in advance – for an instant fix. When counting the calories you need to be strict with portion sizes, dividing them into individual glasses or bowls, and top with one of the many low-fat options such as flavoured or plain yogurt, fromage frais or readymade low-fat custard, obviously taking these extras into account when totting up the calories.

Should you want a more substantial pudding, check out the recipes in the Entertaining section for further ideas.

Chocolate meringue Yule log

SERVES 8
PER SERVING
(APPROXIMATELY):
168 KCAL/2.3G FAT
PREPARATION TIME:
10 MINUTES
COOKING TIME:
30 MINUTES

4 egg whites
175g (6oz) caster sugar
1 teaspoon vanilla essence
300ml (½ pint) Total 0% fat
    Greek yogurt
6 servings Valrhona Chocolate
    Mousse (see recipe, page
    208)
or
225g (8oz) virtually fat free
    chocolate mousse
cocoa powder to dust

Meringue roulade makes an impressive low-fat dessert that can be made a day in advance or stored frozen. This must be the low-fat birthday cake of all time!

1 Preheat the oven to 170C, 350F, Gas Mark 3.
2 Lightly grease and line a large Swiss roll tin with baking parchment.
3 Whisk the egg whites in a dry clean bowl until stiff. Continue whisking, adding the sugar a dessertspoon at a time, allowing 10 seconds between each addition, until all of the sugar is added.
4 Add the vanilla and carefully fold into the mixture using a metal spoon. Pour the mixture into the prepared tin and level off with a palette knife. Bake in the oven for 15 minutes.
5 Reduce the oven temperature to 150C, 300F, Gas Mark 2 and bake for a further 15 minutes.
6 Turn the meringue out onto a piece of foil and peel away the parchment. Allow to cool.
7 Spread a thin layer of yogurt over the roulade, roll up like a Swiss roll and place on a serving plate.
8 Place the chocolate mousse inside a piping bag containing a star shape nozzle and pipe a lattice design across the top.
9 Just before serving, dust with cocoa powder.

Cinnamon and lemon prunes with saffron fromage frais

These prunes make a really tasty low-fat breakfast as well as a tempting dessert. Try them with muesli and low-fat yogurt – simply delicious.

1 Remove the stones from the prunes by squeezing them through the top of the fruit. Place the prunes in a saucepan.

2 Using a zester, zest the lemon into the saucepan, then cut the lemon in half and squeeze the juice into the pan.

3 Snap the cinnamon in half and add to the pan. Add the sugar and sufficient water to just cover, place on a low heat to simmer gently for 20 minutes.

4 Place the saffron and wine in a separate pan and simmer until the wine has almost evaporated. Scrape out and mix into the fromage frais, adding sugar to taste.

5 Serve the prunes hot or cold with a spoonful of fromage frais and a dusting of icing sugar.

SERVES 4
PER SERVING:
136 KCAL/0.2G FAT
PREPARATION TIME:
5 MINUTES
COOKING TIME:
20 MINUTES

225g (8oz) Agen or large prunes
1 lemon
1 cinnamon stick
2 tablespoons soft brown sugar
good pinch of saffron
½ wine glass white wine
300ml (½ pint) virtually fat free
    Normandy fromage frais
icing sugar to dust

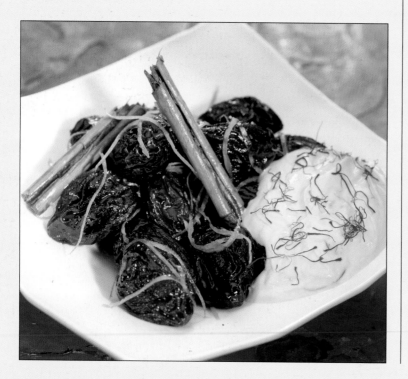

Mango and white rum ice

SERVES 4
PER SERVING:
134 KCAL/0.15G FAT
PREPARATION TIME:
15 MINUTES
COOKING TIME:
10 MINUTES
FREEZING TIME:
12 HOURS

50g (2oz) caster sugar
2 large ripe mangoes
12 pink peppercorns
grated fresh nutmeg
2 tablespoons white rum
1 egg white
fresh mint to decorate

Refreshing and tangy, this fruity iced dessert will round off any meal, especially one containing highly spiced or highly flavoured foods. If you wish, you can omit the alcohol or substitute with a cordial such as elderflower.

1 In a small saucepan dissolve the sugar in 300ml (½ pint) water and bring to the boil. Remove from the heat and allow to cool.
2 Peel the mangoes and remove the flesh from the stone. Place in a food processor, add the peppercorns and a little grated nutmeg and blend until smooth.
3 Mix the fruit purée with the cooled syrup and rum and pour into a shallow freezer container. Cover and freeze for 3 hours until mushy.
4 Remove from the freezer and break up with a fork.
5 Whisk the egg white until stiff. Fold into the loosened mixture and return to the freezer until firm, ideally overnight.
6 Twenty minutes before serving, remove from the freezer and place in the refrigerator to allow it to soften slightly.
7 Serve in a frosted glass decorated with fresh mint.

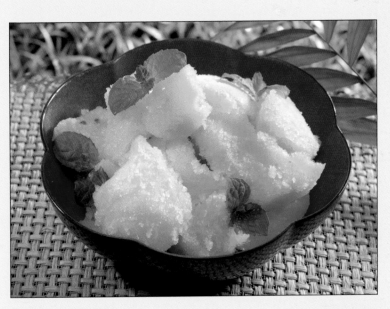

Chestnut meringue roulade

Meringue roulade makes an impressive low-fat dessert that can be made a day in advance or stored frozen. The chopped chestnuts give both added flavour and a crunchy texture. As chestnuts are the only nuts low in fat, this combination offers a tasty treat for all.

1 Preheat the oven to 170C, 350F, Gas Mark 3. Lightly grease and line a large Swiss roll tin with baking parchment.
2 Whisk the egg whites in a dry clean bowl until stiff. Continue whisking, adding the sugar a dessertspoon at a time, allowing 10 seconds between each addition, until all of the sugar is added.
3 Add the vanilla and chestnuts and carefully fold into the mixture using a metal spoon.
4 Pour the mixture into the prepared tin and level off with a palette knife. Bake in the oven for 15 minutes.
5 Reduce the oven temperature to 150C, 300F, Gas Mark 2 and bake for a further 15 minutes.
6 Turn the meringue out onto a piece of foil and peel away the parchment. Allow to cool.
7 In a small bowl mix together the yogurt and chestnut purée, then spread a thin layer over the roulade. Roll up like a Swiss roll and place on a serving plate, decorated with fresh fruit.

SERVES 8
PER SERVING:
112 KCAL/0.3G FAT
PREPARATION TIME:
10 MINUTES
COOKING TIME:
30 MINUTES

4 egg whites
175g (6oz) caster sugar
1 teaspoon vanilla essence
3 tablespoons chopped chestnuts
300ml ($\frac{1}{2}$ pint) Total 0% fat Greek yogurt
2 tablespoons chestnut purée
fresh fruit to decorate

Fresh fruit salad verde

SERVES 4
PER SERVING:
100 KCAL/0.4G FAT
PREPARATION TIME:
10 MINUTES

zest and juice of 2 limes

2 Granny Smith apples

3 kiwi fruit

4 ripe greengage plums, stoned
and sliced

small bunch white seedless
grapes, de-stalked

2 star fruit, sliced

2 teaspoons finely chopped
fresh ginger

1 tablespoon crème de menthe
liqueur

sugar to taste

fresh mint to decorate

Not only does this fruit salad look healthy but it also tastes equally as good. Substitute one or more of the fruits with fresh melon to suit your taste.

1 Place the lime juice and zest in a mixing bowl. Core the apples and slice directly into the bowl to prevent the apples discolouring.
2 Prepare the kiwi by removing the outer skin with a sharp knife; cut the flesh into small slices or sticks and place in the bowl with the plums and remaining fruit.
3 In a small bowl combine the ginger and liqueur then pour onto the salad. Add a little sugar if necessary and chill until required.
4 Serve in tall glasses with a little 0% fat Greek yogurt.

Lime cheesecake ice cream

Light evaporated milk forms the base to this luxurious creamy dessert. It is very important that the milk is completely chilled overnight in order to achieve the thick foam once whisked.

1 Finely grate the lime zest from all four limes into a mixing bowl and add the evaporated milk. Using an electric mixer, whisk the evaporated milk on high speed until thick and double in volume.

2 Cut the limes in half and squeeze out the juice into a small saucepan.

3 Split the vanilla pod lengthways, using a sharp knife. Scrape out the black seeds from the centre and add to the pan, along with the sugar.

4 Heat gently, stirring until the sugar has dissolved. Whisk the hot syrup into the milk until fully combined.

5 Carefully fold in the fromage frais and Quark and pour into a plastic freezer container. Cover and freeze for 4–5 hours until firm.

6 Remove from the freezer 10 minutes before serving. Serve 2–3 scoops per serving sprinkled with the crushed ginger biscuits.

SERVES 6
PER SERVING:
150 KCAL / 1.3G FAT
PREPARATION TIME:
15 MINUTES
COOKING TIME:
5 MINUTES
FREEZING TIME:
4–5 HOURS

4 large limes
2 × 170g cans light evaporated milk, chilled overnight
1 vanilla pod
75g (3oz) caster sugar
225g (8oz) virtually fat free fromage frais
115g (4oz) Quark (low-fat cheese)
3 × 90% fat free ginger biscuits, crushed

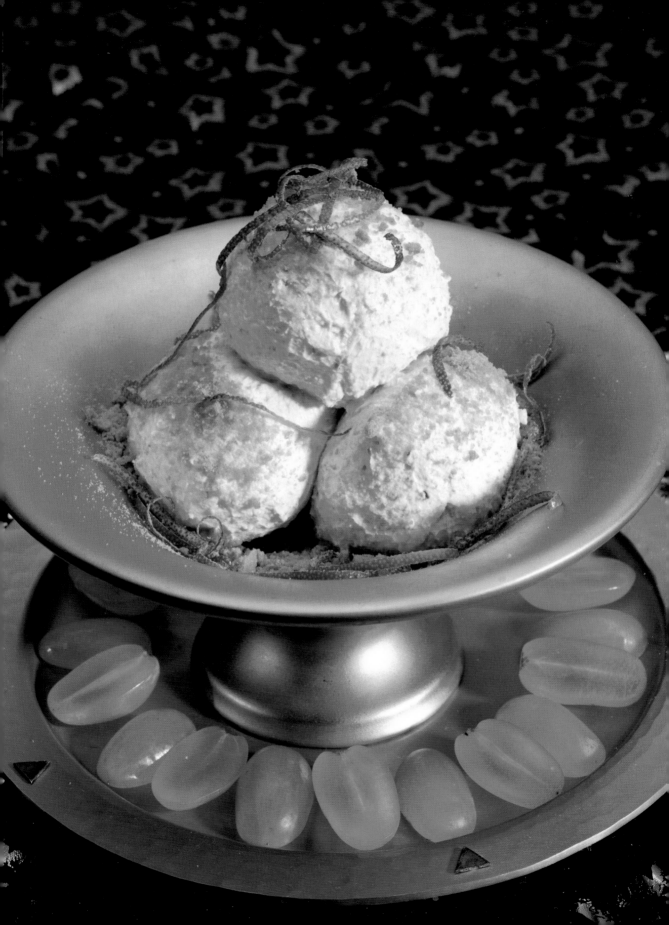

Burgundy poached peaches with strawberry salsa

Turn a simple fruit into an explosion of flavours with this classic combination of red wine and fresh fruit. White flesh peaches tend to be sweeter than the other varieties.

1 In a saucepan combine the wine, orange zest and juice, cardamom seeds and sugar. Bring to the boil then reduce the heat to a gentle simmer.

2 Half-fill a separate pan with water and bring to the boil. With a slotted spoon carefully add the peaches and cook for 2–3 minutes.

3 Remove them from the pan and place immediately into cold water. Carefully peel away the outer skin and place them in the wine mixture. Cook gently for 10–12 minutes until just tender against the point of a knife.

4 Remove the peaches from the pan and place in a serving dish.

5 Place the wine back on the heat and simmer until the liquid has reduced to a thick syrup. Add the chopped strawberries and spoon over the cooked peaches.

6 Decorate with fresh mint and serve hot or cold with low-fat fromage frais.

SERVES 4
PER SERVING:
151 KCAL/0.2G FAT
PREPARATION TIME:
10 MINUTES
COOKING TIME:
20 MINUTES

450ml (¾ pint) Burgundy wine
zest and juice of 1 orange
8 cardamom pods, crushed
    seeds removed
2 tablespoons Muscovado sugar
4 large white flesh peaches
225g (8oz) fresh strawberries,
    hulled and chopped
fresh mint to decorate

Orange Panna Cotta with fresh orange

SERVES 4

PER SERVING:
75 KCAL/0.4G FAT

PREPARATION TIME:
5 MINUTES

COOKING TIME:
10 MINUTES

300ml (1/2 pint) skimmed milk

3 × 35g sachets orange Quick Jel

fine zest of 1 large orange

300ml (1/2 pint) low-fat natural yogurt

icing sugar to dust

Panna Cotta is an Italian dessert usually made by adding a setting agent to warmed flavoured single cream, resulting in a smooth blancmange-like texture. Our low-fat version is certainly easier to prepare and you will not believe this smooth, luxurious treat.

1 Pour the milk into a saucepan and sprinkle the Quick Jel over. Heat gently, stirring continuously, until the mixture starts to thicken. Simmer for 2–3 minutes.

2 Remove from the heat and stir in the orange zest. Allow to cool slightly, then stir in the yogurt until smooth.

3 Pour into 4 individual moulds or 1 large one and refrigerate overnight or until set.

4 Cut away the peel from the zested orange and split the orange into segments.

5 To turn out the Panna Cotta, dip the mould quickly into a bowl of boiling water, place an upturned serving plate on top and quickly flip the mould and plate over. Remove the mould and decorate with orange segments and a dusting of icing sugar.

Raspberry bavarois

There are many different types of fromage frais and low-fat yogurts available that can be used for this type of recipe. Choose good-quality varieties that tend to have a rich texture and not such sharp flavours. Make this recipe in advance and store refrigerated until ready to serve.

1 Soak the gelatine in cold water for 2–3 minutes until it becomes soft. Place it in a bowl and heat it either over a pan of boiling water or in a microwave for 1 minute until liquid.
2 Add the fromage frais and Grenadine and mix together thoroughly. Carefully fold in the raspberries with a little sugar to taste and blend again until combined.
3 Whisk the egg whites until stiff and fold into the mixture.
4 Spoon into individual glasses or place in a glass bowl and decorate with extra raspberries, blackberries and mint leaves.

SERVES 4
PER SERVING:
107 KCAL/0.4G FAT
PREPARATION TIME:
5 MINUTES
COOKING TIME:
10 MINUTES

6 sheets leaf gelatine
450g (16oz) virtually fat free
    Normandy fromage frais
2 tablespoons Grenadine
275g (10oz) fresh raspberries
caster sugar to taste
3 egg whites
a few raspberries, blackberries
    and mint leaves to decorate

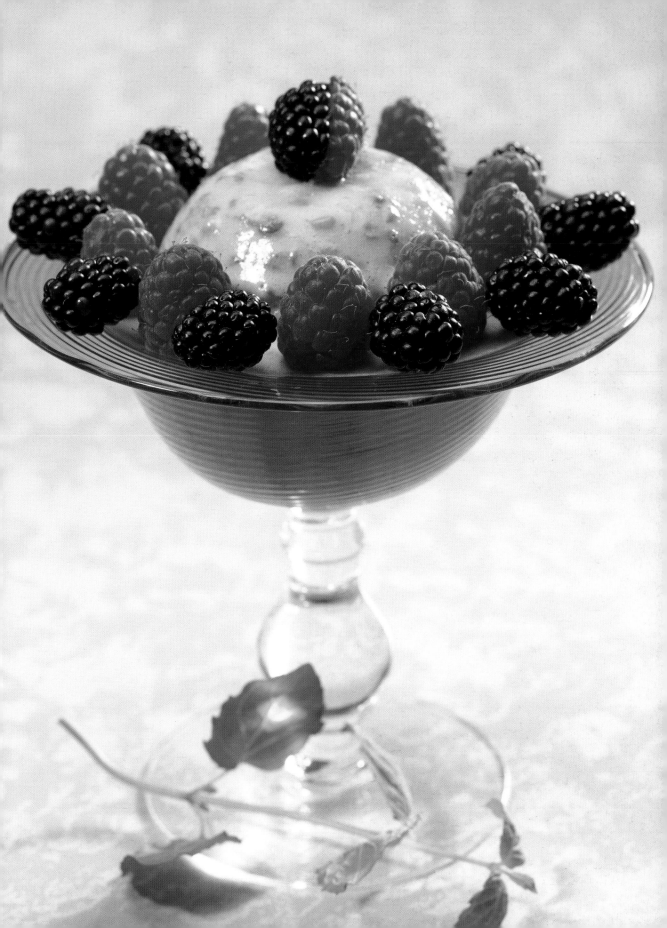

Kiwi and passion fruit salad with balsamic dressing

An unusual combination of sweet and savoury. If you find the balsamic too strong, try replacing with mild fruit vinegar such as cherry or raspberry.

1 Prepare the kiwi by removing the outer skin with a sharp knife. Cut the flesh into small slices and place in a bowl.
2 Cut the passion fruit in half, scoop out the seeds with a teaspoon and add to the kiwi.
3 In a small bowl combine the lime juice and zest with the balsamic vinegar, adding a little sugar if necessary. Arrange on a plate and chill until required.

SERVES 1
PER SERVING:
62 KCAL/0.4GFAT
PREPARATION TIME:
5 MINUTES

1 kiwi fruit
1 passion fruit
zest and juice of 1 lime
2–3 teaspoons balsamic vinegar
sugar to taste

Entertaining

Once you get into the routine of low-fat cooking you will probably find the need to expand your talents to more challenging treats or surprise guests with a low-fat creation of your own. Use this section alongside your diet recipes to add variation for all the family.

Starters

Designed as a little tasty intro, a starter can act as a useful low-calorie filler, enabling you to reduce the size of the courses to follow. Fruit, salads and fresh soups are always simple options, but sometimes we like to stretch to something a little more unusual, especially when entertaining guests.

Many of these substantial starter recipes will double up as light lunches with the addition of a salad or bread where appropriate.

Roasted pepper tarts

*Simple and stylish, these attractive tarts make a great entertaining
starter or buffet party food. Vary the filling, using different
combinations of cooked or roasted vegetables.*

1 Preheat the oven to 190C, 375F, Gas Mark 5.
2 Cut the peppers in half, remove the seeds and place face down
   on a non-stick baking sheet. Roast in the top of the oven for
   20–30 minutes until soft. Remove from the oven and place
   inside a plastic food bag. Seal the bag and leave to cool. Peel
   the cooled peppers and roughly chop.
2 Stack the filo pastry sheets on top of each other. Using scissors,
   cut the stack into 6 equal square sections, so that you end up
   with 36 individual squares.
3 Take 6 non-stick individual tartlet tins, 10cm (4in) in diameter.
   In each tin, place 6 individual pastry squares in layers, placing
   the squares at slight angles to each other and brushing with
   beaten egg white in between each layer.
4 Bake in the oven for 8–10 minutes until crisp and golden. Allow
   to cool.
5 To make the filling, in a mixing bowl combine the chopped
   peppers with the remaining ingredients except the olives and
   season well. Spoon the mixture into the baked shells and return
   to the oven to warm through.
6 Garnish each tart with half a black olive. Serve warm with a
   variety of freshly prepared salads.

MAKES 6
PER TART:
94 KCAL / 1.7G FAT
PREPARATION TIME:
40 MINUTES
COOKING TIME:
20 MINUTES

3 red peppers
6 sheets filo pastry
   (30 × 20cm / 12 × 8in)
1 egg white, beaten
handful of fresh basil leaves
1 teaspoon vegetable bouillon
   stock powder
2 tablespoons tomato passata
salt and freshly ground black
   pepper
3 black olives to garnish

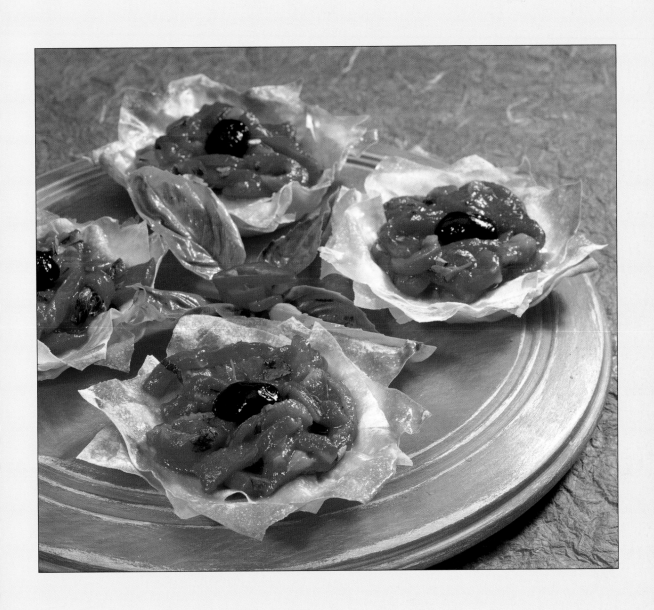

Thai cod fritters with tomato dipping sauce

This spicy fish starter can be made in advance and reheated in a warm oven. It is important to add plenty of seasoning to bring out the full flavour of the spices.

1 Poach the cod in the vegetable stock until just cooked and allow to cool.

2 In a medium saucepan combine the milk, onion, chilli and lemongrass and bring to the boil. Slake the cornflour with a little cold water and add to the pan, stirring continuously as the mixture thickens. Reduce the heat and simmer for 3–4 minutes.

3 Pour the mixture into a bowl and allow to cool. Mix in the cod and coriander, season well with salt and freshly ground black pepper, then refrigerate for 1 hour.

4 To make the dipping sauce, combine all the ingredients, season with salt and black pepper and place in a small bowl.

5 Remove the cod mixture from the refrigerator. Preheat a non-stick frying pan. Drop tablespoon-sized amounts of the mixture into the pan and dry-fry for 2–3 minutes on each side.

6 Allow 2 per person and serve with salad leaves and the dipping sauce.

SERVES 6
PER SERVING:
75 KCAL/1.1G FAT
PREPARATION TIME:
10 MINUTES
COOKING TIME:
20 MINUTES
CHILLING TIME 1 HOUR

115g (4oz) thick cod fillet
150ml (1/4 pint) vegetable stock
150ml (1/4 pint) skimmed milk
1 red onion, finely chopped
1 small red chilli, seeded and finely chopped
2 teaspoons lemongrass, finely chopped
1 tablespoon cornflour
1 tablespoon chopped fresh coriander
salt and freshly ground black pepper

for the dipping sauce
150ml (1/4 pint) tomato passata
1 tablespoon hot mango chutney
1 tablespoon light soy sauce
1 teaspoon finely grated lime zest
salt and freshly ground black pepper

Caramelised onion tarts

MAKES 6
PER TART 211 KCAL/6G FAT
PREPARATION TIME:
40 MINUTES
COOKING TIME:
20 MINUTES

6 sheets filo pastry
   (30cm × 20cm/12 × 8in)
1 egg white, beaten
1kg (2lb) onions, sliced
4 garlic cloves, crushed
1 teaspoon caster sugar
2 eggs
1 tablespoon fresh thyme leaves
2 teaspoons vegetable bouillon
   stock powder
115g (4oz) low-fat Cheddar
   cheese
1 tablespoon chopped fresh
   chives
salt and freshly ground black
   pepper

Caramelising onions gives a rich colour as well as a sweet nutty flavour. As the pastry is very thin, assemble at the last minute before the final cooking.

1 Preheat the oven to 190C, 375F, Gas Mark 5.
2 Stack the filo pastry sheets on top of each other. Using scissors, cut the stack into 6 equal square sections so that you end up with 36 individual squares.
3 Take 6 non-stick individual tartlet tins, 10cm (4in) in diameter. In each tin, place 6 individual pastry squares in layers, placing the squares at slight angles to each other with beaten egg white brushed in between each layer.
4 Bake in the oven for 5 minutes until dry. Allow to cool.
5 To make the filling, preheat a non-stick frying pan until hot. Add the onions, garlic and caster sugar and dry-fry for 4–5 minutes until they start to caramelise and turn brown.
6 In a mixing bowl beat the eggs, add the thyme, stock powder and cheese. Quickly mix in the onion mixture and the chopped chives, seasoning with salt and freshly ground black pepper. Spoon into the pastry cases and bake in the oven for 10–15 minutes until set.
7 Serve warm with a mixed leaf salad.

Chicken liver and bacon satés with oyster sauce

Canapés and nibbles are usually pastry based with rich creamy fillings. Try this Chinese twist on liver and bacon served hot with salad or just as simple finger food.

1 Drain the chicken livers well and cut into bite-size pieces, discarding any dark or fatty parts. Season with salt and freshly ground black pepper.

2 Cut the bacon into 8 evenly sized strips. Take 8 cocktail sticks and thread the bacon like a concertina onto the sticks, placing a piece of chicken liver in between each fold. Place in a shallow dish.

3 Combine the remaining ingredients and pour over the meat, cover and refrigerate until required.

4 Cook under a hot preheated grill for 1–2 minutes, depending on personal taste. Serve hot.

SERVES 4
PER SERVING:
129 KCAL / 2.9G FAT
PREPARATION TIME:
15 MINUTES
COOKING TIME:
2–3 MINUTES

225g (8oz) chicken livers, soaked in milk for approx. 30 minutes
4 lean rashers smoked or plain rindless bacon
3 tablespoon Chinese oyster sauce
2 tablespoons clear honey
1 tablespoon Chinese hoisin sauce
2–3 drops Tabasco
salt and freshly ground black pepper

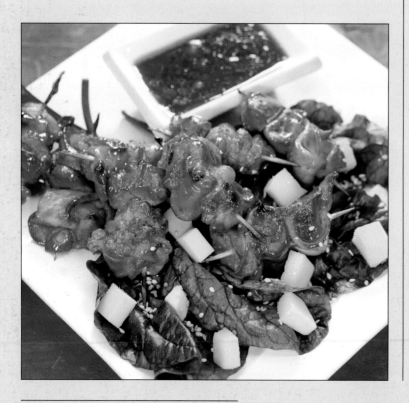

Baked aubergines

SERVES 4
PER SERVING:
91 KCAL / 5.8G FAT
PREPARATION TIME:
10 MINUTES
COOKING TIME:
60 MINUTES

2 medium aubergines
4 rashers lean smoked bacon,
   diced
6–8 large basil leaves
2 garlic cloves, finely chopped
2 tablespoons good-quality red
   wine vinegar
2 tomatoes skinned, seeded and
   diced
salt and freshly ground black
   pepper
chopped fresh parsley and salad
   to garnish

1 Preheat the oven to 180C, 350F, Gas Mark 4.
2 Slice the aubergines in half lengthways and place in a shallow
   ovenproof dish. Using a sharp knife, make incisions across the
   cut side of each aubergine to leave a crosshatch pattern.
3 Tear the basil leaves into small pieces and mix together with
   the bacon and garlic in a small bowl. Press the mixture into the
   incisions, distributing the mixture evenly. Season with salt and
   pepper and drizzle with the vinegar.
4 Place in the preheated oven and bake for 1 hour or until soft.
5 Remove from the oven and cover with the diced tomato.
6 Serve hot or cold sprinkled with chopped fresh parsley on a
   salad garnish.

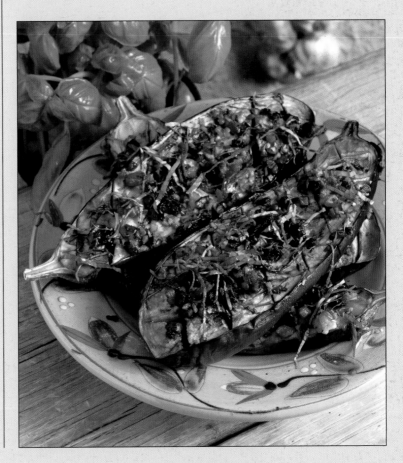

Hors d'oeuvres au aïoli

Hors d'oeuvres can vary from thin pieces of toasted bread topped with pâté or vegetable pastes to more delicate terrines and fish dishes. A selection of flavoursome vegetables lightly cooked with a garlic dipping sauce makes an ideal introduction to French cuisine. Aïoli is traditionally made using a large quantity of egg yolks and olive oil.

1 Cook the vegetables individually in a pan of boiling salted water until just tender. Drain and arrange in colourful clusters around the outside of a serving plate.
2 In a small bowl combine all the sauce ingredients, seasoning well with salt and freshly ground black pepper. Place in the centre of the plate and serve either hot or cold.

See photograph on page 166.

SERVES 4
PER SERVING:
93 KCAL/0.8G FAT
PREPARATION TIME:
10 MINUTES
COOKING TIME:
20 MINUTES

115g (4oz) French beans, trimmed
115g (4oz) small carrots
4 baby courgettes
8 cherry tomatoes
1 sweet potato, peeled and cut into wedges

for the aïoli sauce
175g (6oz) virtually fat free fromage frais
2 tablespoons cider vinegar
1 tablespoon lime juice
$1/4$ teaspoon ground turmeric
2 teaspoons sugar
2 garlic cloves, crushed
salt and freshly ground black pepper

Mediterranean courgette boats

SERVES 4
PER SERVING:
97 KCAL/3.4G FAT
PREPARATION TIME:
15 MINUTES
COOKING TIME:
35 MINUTES

8 medium courgettes
1 small red onion, finely
   chopped
2 garlic cloves, crushed
1 red and 1 yellow pepper,
   seeded and finely diced
115g (4oz) chestnut mushrooms,
   finely chopped
1–2 tablespoons tomato purée
2 tablespoons chopped fresh
   basil
salt and freshly ground black
   pepper
25g (1oz) Parmesan cheese,
   grated

Make these cheesy vegetable boats in advance and cook when required. You may find the need to add a little water to the vegetable mixture, depending on the strength of the tomato purée.

1 Preheat the oven to 200C, 400F, Gas Mark 6.
2 Slice the courgettes down the centre and, using a teaspoon, carefully remove as much of the flesh from the centre of each half. Chop the flesh and set aside. Season the courgette shells with salt and freshly ground black pepper and place side by side in an ovenproof dish.
3 Preheat a non-stick pan. Dry-fry the onion, garlic and courgettes for 2–3 minutes until soft. Add the pepper and mushrooms, continuing to cook over a high heat. Remove from the heat and stir in the tomato purée and chopped basil.
4 Pile the mixture into the courgette shells and top with the Parmesan cheese.
5 Bake in the preheated oven for 20–25 minutes until the shells are cooked. Serve hot or cold.

See photograph on page 166.

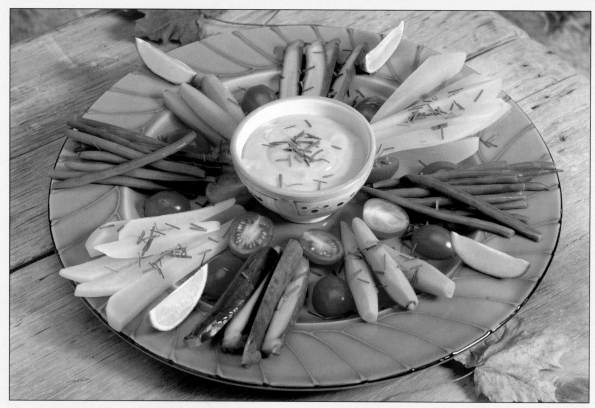

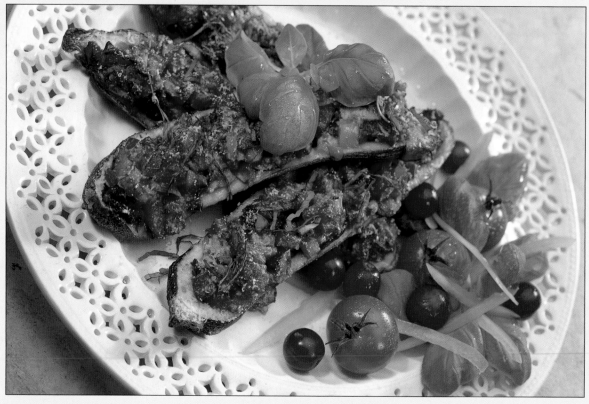

Smoked mackerel and sweet mustard pâté

SERVES 4
PER SERVING:
229 KCAL/18G FAT
PREPARATION TIME:
15 MINUTES

225g (8oz) smoked mackerel
    fillets
1 tablespoon coarse grain
    mustard
115g (4oz) Quark (low-fat
    cheese)
1 tablespoon chopped fresh
    parsley
juice of $\frac{1}{2}$ lemon
salt and freshly ground black
    pepper
salad to garnish

1 Using a fork, break up the mackerel fillets in a small bowl. Add
   the mustard, Quark, parsley and lemon juice. Mix well and
   season with salt and freshly ground black pepper.
2 Press the mixture into 4 ramekin dishes and smooth the tops
   over with a knife.
3 Refrigerate until ready to serve.

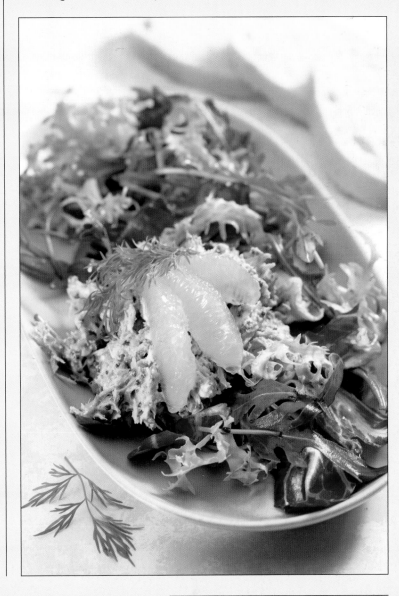

Top left: *Hors d'oeuvres au aïoli*

Left: *Mediterranean courgette boats*

Sundried tomato hummus with roasted summer vegetables

Hummus is a garlic spiked chickpea paste usually made with a large quantity of oil as well as high-fat chickpeas. The tomatoes add colour and a sweet flavour, making it much lighter to eat. Squeezing a little fresh lemon over adds that extra little touch. Stored refrigerated, it will keep for 5 days.

1 Preheat the oven to 200C, 400F, Gas Mark 6.
2 Place all the vegetables into a roasting tray and drizzle with the soy sauce. Roast in the top of the oven for 20–25 minutes, turning occasionally. Allow to cool.
3 In a saucepan, heat the milk with the dried tomatoes and garlic. Reduce the heat and simmer for 8–10 minutes until the tomatoes have softened. Allow to cool.
4 Drain and rinse the chickpeas and place in a food processor. Pour in the milk mixture and process until smooth. Season with lots of salt and freshly ground black pepper, add the lemon juice, then blend again to combine. Adjust the consistency with a little extra milk if required.
5 Arrange the cooled vegetables on a serving plate, placing a spoonful of hummus in the centre.

See photograph on page 170.

SERVES 4
PER SERVING:
230 KCAL / 6.2G FAT
PREPARATION TIME:
20 MINUTES
COOKING TIME:
25 MINUTES

for the roasted vegetables
2 baby courgettes, sliced
2 red and 2 yellow peppers,
    seeded and cut into chunks
3 baby leeks, sliced
8 small vine tomatoes
1 teaspoon chopped fresh
    rosemary
handful of fresh basil leaves
2 tablespoons light soy sauce

for the hummus
3–4 pieces sundried tomato
    (non-oil type)
2 garlic cloves, crushed
300ml ($\frac{1}{2}$ pint) skimmed milk
1 × 425g (15oz) can chickpeas
    with no added salt or sugar
juice of 1 lemon
salt and freshly ground black
    pepper

Salt cod and red pepper brandade

SERVES 6
PER SERVING:
201 KCAL/1.1G FAT
(EXCLUDING FRENCH BREAD)
PREPARATION TIME:
2 DAYS' SOAKING
COOKING TIME:
35 MINUTES

700g (1lb 9oz) salt cod
600ml (1 pint) skimmed milk
1 bay leaf
3 red peppers
2 garlic cloves
juice of 1 lemon
coarsely ground black pepper
1 tablespoon chopped fresh
    parsley or coriander to
    garnish
toasted French bread to serve

1 Preheat the oven to 200C, 400F, Gas Mark 6.
2 Soak the cod in cold water for 2 days, changing the water every 12 hours.
3 Place the fish in a shallow pan containing the milk and bay leaf and poach gently until cooked. Allow to cool.
4 Cut the peppers in half, remove and discard the central core and seeds and place on a non-stick roasting tray with the garlic. Cook in the preheated oven for 25 minutes until they start to blister. Remove from the oven and place the hot peppers in a plastic food bag and seal – this will make it easier to remove the skins. Allow to cool.
5 Remove the fish from the cooking liquor and strain the liquid through a sieve into a jug. Flake the fish, removing any skin and bones, and place in a food processor with the lemon and the garlic from the roasting tray. Process on high, adding the milk gradually to create a thick paste, season with black pepper and spread onto toasted French bread.
6 Remove the peppers from the bag and carefully peel away the skins. Slice into thick strips and arrange on top of the brandade. Sprinkle with parsley or coriander and servewith toasted French bread.

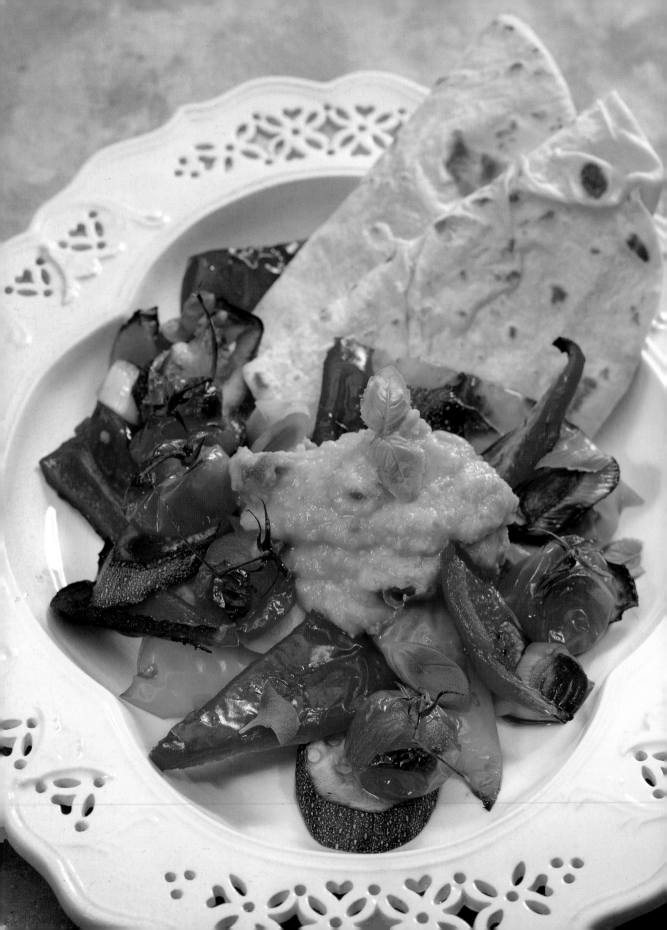

Pink grapefruit and grenadine cocktail

SERVES 4
PER SERVING:
93 KCAL/0.2G FAT
PREPARATION TIME:
10 MINUTES
COOKING TIME:
10 MINUTES

4 medium pink grapefruit
1 tablespoon soft brown sugar
zest and juice of 1 lime
2 teaspoons finely chopped
   fresh ginger
2 tablespoons Grenadine
mint leaves or lime zest to
   garnish

Grenadine is syrup made from the pomegranate fruit. Being red in colour it has a magical effect on fruits and salads giving them an exotic appeal.

1 Prepare the grapefruit by slicing away the skin and pith with a sharp knife to reveal the fruit. Cut in between the thin connecting membrane, separating and removing each segment into a mixing bowl. Sprinkle the sugar, lime and ginger over and spoon into serving glasses.

2 Divide the Grenadine between the 4 glasses and garnish with fresh mint or lime zest.

3 Serve chilled as a light starter or alternatively a refreshing simple dessert.

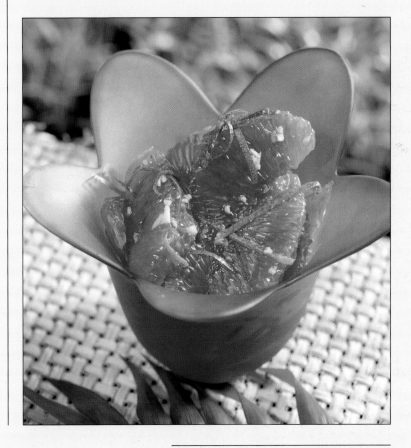

Left: *Sundried tomato hummus with roasted summer vegetables*

Griddled Madagascan prawns with orange and tomato glaze

Large prawns make a good starter or buffet party food. This recipe also works well with scallops or dense fish such as monkfish or fresh tuna.

1 Peel the prawns and remove the intestinal vein by carefully making a shallow cut along the back of the prawn to reveal a dark vein. This will easily pull away from the main body of the prawn.
2 Thread the prawns onto skewers and place in the bottom of a shallow dish.
3 Combine the remaining ingredients and pour over the prawns. Allow to marinate in the refrigerator for 2–3 hours.
4 Preheat a non-stick griddle pan until hot. Place the prawns in the pan and cook for 2–3 minutes on each side, basting with the marinade during cooking.
5 Serve immediately on a bed of crisp green salad.

SERVES 6
PER SERVING:
41 KCAL/1G FAT
PREPARATION TIME:
20 MINUTES
COOKING TIME:
2-3 MINUTES

25–30 Madagascan or jumbo prawns
4 tablespoons freshly squeezed orange juice
1 tablespoon light soy sauce
1 tablespoon chopped fresh tarragon
150ml ($\frac{1}{4}$ pint) tomato passata
2 garlic cloves, crushed

Melon and mango towers

SERVES 4
PER SERVING:
175 KCAL/3G FAT
PREPARATION TIME:
10 MINUTES
COOKING TIME:
10 MINUTES

selection of assorted melons
   (water, Ogen, Charentais,
   cantaloupe)
2 ripe mangoes
3 tablespoons mild mango
   chutney
1 × 2.5cm (1in) piece ginger,
   finely chopped
1 tablespoon light brown sugar

Simple, stylish appetisers are always welcome before a main meal.
This recipe uses very few ingredients, yet it looks very impressive as
a starter or even an alternative fruit dessert.

1 Prepare the melons by slicing down the sides of the fruit to give
   long thin pieces of fruit. Then, using a large pastry cutter,
   approximately 6cm (3in) in diameter, cut out approximately
   12–16 discs of the fruit, depending on the size of the fruits.
   Using a smaller cutter, 2.5cm (1in) in diameter, remove the
   centre from each disc and reserve.
2 Peel the mangoes and again slice away the flesh in long pieces
   around the shape of the inner stone.
3 On a serving dish place 4 circles of melon side by side and
   spread lightly with the mango chutney. Add slices of mango,
   spread with the chutney, and then more melon. Keep building
   until the stacks are 3–4 melon slices deep.
4 Chop the remaining melon and mango, saving 4 inner discs for
   the tops. Combine the chopped fruits with the ginger and
   sugar, place in the centre of each tower and top with the
   reserved discs.
5 Chill until required.

Blinis with smoked salmon and horseradish cream

Blinis are light batter pancakes often used as a canapé or starter to serve as a base for salmon or caviar. Our low-fat version can be made in different sizes to suit. For a neat, uniform look use a round pastry cutter to trim them to equal size.

1 Warm the milk to a temperature that's no more than hand hot. Add the yeast and whisk well.

2 Combine the flours in a mixing bowl, add the egg yolk and fromage frais, then, using a whisk, gradually pour in the milk, beating the mixture to a smooth, lump-free batter. Allow to stand and prove for 30 minutes.

3 Whisk the egg whites with a pinch of salt to stiff peaks, then carefully fold into the batter with a metal spoon.

4 Preheat a non-stick frying pan, then lightly oil the pan, removing the oil with kitchen paper.

5 Spoon tablespoons of the mixture separately into the pan and cook for 1 minute, flip over and cook the other side for a further 2 minutes. Allow to cool on a wire rack.

6 Place the blinis on a serving plate. Drape the smoked salmon on top.

7 Mix together the fromage frais and horseradish, seasoning well with salt and freshly ground black pepper, and spoon on top. Garnish with fresh dill.

SERVES 6
PER SERVING:
226 KCAL/2.7G FAT
PREPARATION TIME:
20 MINUTES
COOKING TIME:
10 MINUTES

for the blinis
300ml (½ pint) skimmed milk
15g (½oz) fresh or dried yeast
175g (6oz) plain flour
75g (3oz) buckwheat flour
1 egg yolk
75g (3oz) virtually fat free fromage frais
4 egg whites
pinch of salt
a little vegetable oil for the pan

for the topping
115g (4oz) smoked salmon
4 tablespoons virtually fat free fromage frais
1 teaspoon horseradish sauce
salt and freshly ground black pepper
sprigs of fresh dill to garnish

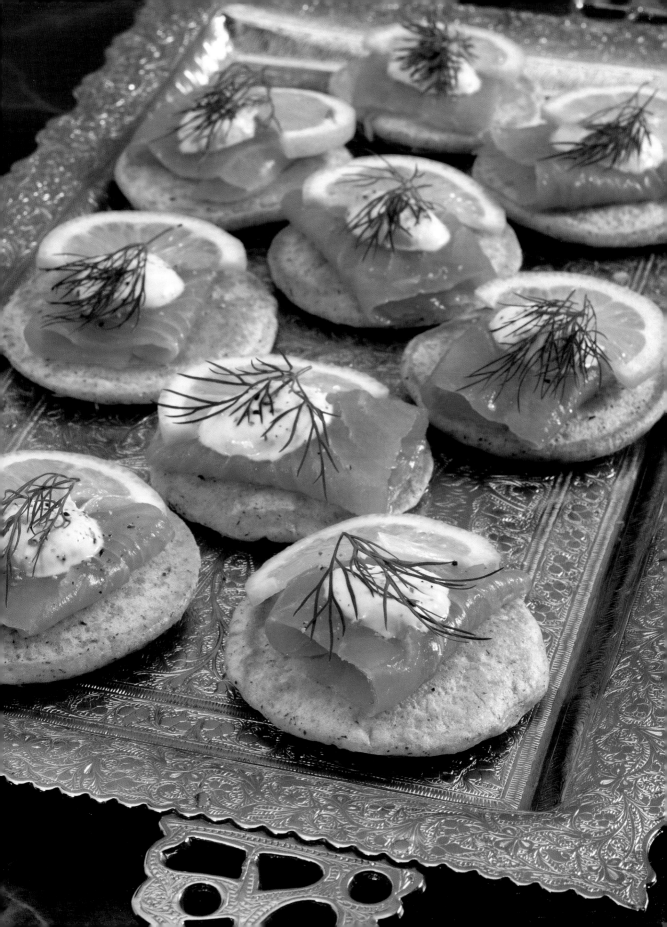

Main courses

Select from light flavoursome dishes to more elaborate creations, giving you the option to design a menu suitable for your requirements. Mix and match the accompaniments, taking into account the calorie and fat content to achieve a well-balanced meal.

Seared beef with chilli bean salad and radish salsa

SERVES 4
PER SERVING:
491 KCAL/16G FAT
PREPARATION TIME:
10 MINUTES
COOKING TIME:
10 MINUTES

4 lean fillet steaks
225g (8oz) fresh fine green
    beans, cut in half
1 × 450g (16oz) can red kidney
    beans, drained
1 × 450g (16oz) can cannellini
    beans, drained
1 small red onion, finely
    chopped
1 red bullet chilli, finely chopped
6 ripe tomatoes, skinned and
    finely chopped
1 tablespoon finely chopped
    chives
2 teaspoons horseradish sauce
salt and freshly ground black
    pepper

for the salsa
1 bunch of young radishes,
    finely chopped
1 small green pepper, finely
    chopped
1 tablespoon chopped fresh
    mint
1 tablespoon mild mango
    chutney

This chunky bean salad can form the base to many light lunches, not just with beef. Try it with seared lean pork or turkey slices. It also works particularly well with gammon.

1 Season the steaks with salt and freshly ground black pepper and set aside.
2 Cook the green beans in a pan of lightly salted water until tender. Drain, rinse with cold water and place in a bowl containing the drained kidney and cannellini beans. Add the remaining ingredients and season with salt and freshly ground black pepper, mixing them until fully combined.
3 Preheat a non-stick frying pan until hot. Add the steaks, cooking them for 2–3 minutes on both sides. Remove from the pan and allow to rest for 2 minutes on a chopping board.
4 Combine the salsa ingredients and place in a small serving bowl.
5 Divide the bean salad between 4 bowls, slice the beef into thick pieces and arrange on top. Garnish with the salsa.

Sage and onion roast pork

Spring onions form the centre to this traditional roast. Using fresh sage gives a much stronger flavour than using dried, adding depth and a distinctive herb flavour to the finished sauce.

1 Preheat the oven to 200C, 400F, Gas Mark 6.
2 Trim away all the fat from the pork, then weigh the joint to calculate the cooking time and lay out flat on a chopping board. Season well with salt and pepper.
3 Dry-fry the onion in a non-stick pan until soft. Add the apple and sage, stir well then remove from the heat and allow to cool.
4 Place the mixture onto the pork, then lay the spring onions across horizontally. Roll the pork up and tie with string. Place the joint in a roasting tin. Spoon the honey over the pork and pour 300ml (½ pint) stock around the meat. Cover with foil and cook in the oven, allowing 30 minutes per 450g (1lb), plus 30 minutes over.
5 Remove the pork from the tin and allow to rest, keeping it covered with foil.
6 Add the remaining stock and wine to the tin and stir well, picking up the meat juices from the bottom. Pour the mixture into a saucepan and heat.
7 Slake the cornflour with a little cold water and stir into the gravy. Simmer gently to allow the gravy to thicken.
8 Slice the pork and arrange on a serving dish with the accompanying sauce.
9 Serve with potatoes, seasonal vegetables and apple sauce.

SERVES 4
PER SERVING:
559 KCAL/14G FAT
PREPARATION TIME:
20 MINUTES
COOKING TIME:
2 HOURS

1.5kg (3lb) lean pork loin joint, boned
2 onions, finely chopped
1 large cooking apple, peeled and grated
2 tablespoons chopped fresh sage
12 thin spring onions
3 tablespoons clear honey
600ml (1 pint) vegetable stock
1 tablespoon cornflour
1 wine glass white wine
salt and freshly ground black pepper

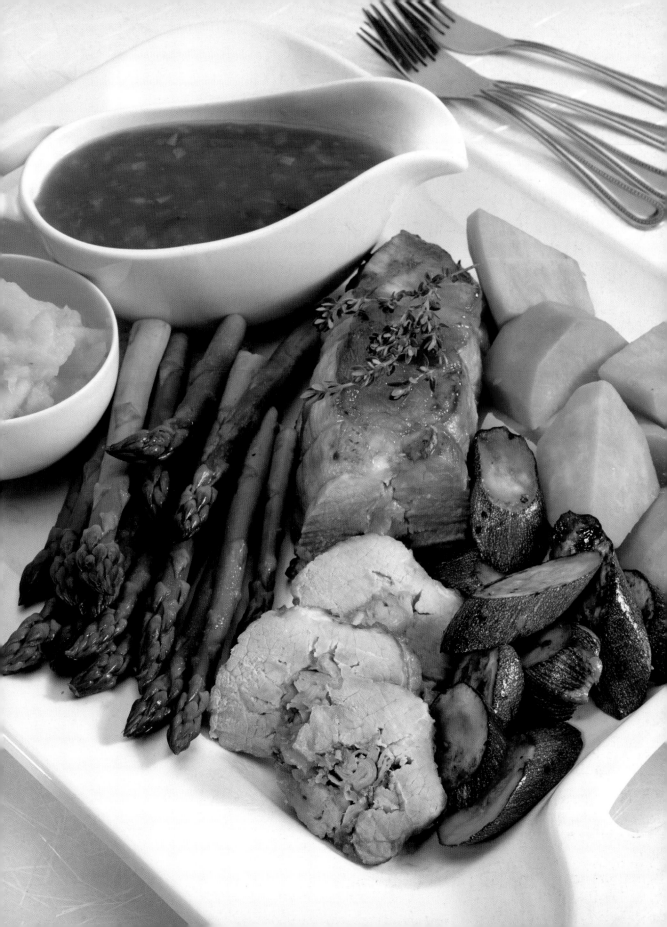

Coconut roasted sea bass wrapped in banana leaves

Toasting the coconut adds a wonderful flavour to this all-in-one fish dish. Using only a small quantity keeps the dish still fairly low in fat, bearing in mind desiccated coconut contains 62% fat. Banana leaves can be found in supermarkets alongside exotic fruit and vegetables and, more recently, in some florists. They are perfect for wrapping around foods for oven roasting since their waxy surface prevents the food from sticking. As well as being attractive, they impart a light, grassy, oriental flavour to the food.

Pre-cooked express rice, available from supermarkets, is a great time-saver and instant accompaniment. Use straight from the packet or jazz it up with herbs.

1 Preheat the oven to 180C, 350F, Gas Mark 4.
2 Wash the fish well inside and out and, using kitchen scissors, trim the fins and tail. Season the inside of the fish with plenty of salt and pepper and lay the lime slices (reserving a few for the garnish) along the length of the inside of the fish.
3 Lay the banana leaf out on a baking tray. Place the rice in a line along one edge, sprinkle with the cardamom seeds and arrange the fish on top.
4 Preheat a non-stick frying pan and dry-fry the coconut over a low heat until lightly toasted. Scatter over the top of the fish and season well with salt and freshly ground black pepper. Place the fresh dill on top, then wrap the banana leaves around the fish, covering as much of the fish as possible (you may need to wrap the head and tail in baking foil).
5 Bake in the oven for 20–25 minutes until just cooked. Remove the foil, if used, and transfer the fish to a serving dish.
6 Garnish with the reserved lime slices and extra fresh dill.

SERVES 6
PER SERVING:
424 KCAL/15G FAT
PREPARATION TIME:
20 MINUTES
COOKING TIME:
30 MINUTES

1.5kg (3lb) sea bass, de-scaled and gutted
2 limes, sliced
1 large or 2 small banana leaves
450g (16oz) [cooked weight] basmati rice
4–5 cardamom pods, crushed and seeds removed
3 tablespoons shredded, desiccated coconut
2–3 sprigs fresh dill
sea salt and freshly ground black pepper

Baked trout with smoked garlic and pesto topping

SERVES 1
PER SERVING:
376 KCAL/12G FAT
PREPARATION TIME:
20 MINUTES
COOKING TIME:
25 MINUTES

1 large trout, gutted
sea salt
1 large sprig fresh rosemary
1 slice of lime
1 smoked garlic clove, finely
    chopped

for the pesto
1 vegetable stock cube
2 good bunches fresh basil
1 tablespoon peeled cooked
    chestnuts
2 teaspoons grated Parmesan
    cheese
salt and freshly ground black
    pepper

Prepare this recipe in advance to allow the flavours of the garlic and pesto to permeate the fish. You will only need 1 tablespoon of pesto for this recipe, but you can freeze the remainder or it will keep in the refrigerator for a few days.

1 Preheat the oven to 200C, 400F, Gas Mark 6.
2 Make the pesto by placing all the ingredients into a liquidiser or food processor and blending until smooth.
3 Rinse the trout well under cold running water. Scrape your finger along the inside of the backbone to remove any traces of blood. Use scissors to trim the tail and cut off all the fins.
4 Place the fish on a baking sheet and slash the top with a sharp knife, making diagonal incisions. Season the inside with sea salt and place a sprig of rosemary, a slice of lime and a little of the chopped garlic inside.
5 Using a pastry brush, spread 1 tablespoon of pesto over the fish, working it down into the incisions.
6 Bake in the oven for 20–25 minutes. Serve hot or cold.

Salmon and broccoli lasagne

This recipe can be made in advance and cooked as required. It is suitable for home freezing.

1 Preheat the oven to 190C, 375F, Gas Mark 5.
2 Cook the broccoli in boiling salted water, drain and set aside.
3 Place the salmon in a saucepan with the milk and cook gently over a low heat for 5–6 minutes. Allow to cool, then lift out the fish onto a plate and flake, removing all skin and bones.
4 Reheat the milk, adding the mustard and stock powder to the saucepan. Slake the cornflour with a little cold water and add to the milk, stirring well to prevent any lumps forming.
5 Add the mushrooms and cheese and mix well. Simmer gently until the sauce is of a coating consistency. Adjust if necessary with a little extra milk or diluted cornflour. Stir in the herbs.
6 Place a thin layer of sauce in the bottom of an ovenproof dish. Cover with sheets of lasagne without overlapping. Add a layer of flaked fish and broccoli then continue layering, ending with the sauce.
7 Bake in the oven for 30–35 minutes until bubbling hot.

SERVES 4
PER SERVING:
658 KCAL/23G FAT
PREPARATION TIME:
5 MINUTES
COOKING TIME:
35 MINUTES

225g (8oz) broccoli, trimmed
4 × 175g (4 × 6oz) salmon fillets
600ml (1 pint) skimmed milk
2 teaspoons Dijon mustard
2 teaspoons vegetable bouillon stock powder
2 tablespoons cornflour
115g (4oz) chestnut mushrooms, sliced
50g (2oz) low-fat Cheddar cheese, grated
1 tablespoon chopped fresh dill
1 tablespoon chopped fresh parsley
225g (8oz) 'no cook' lasagne
salt and freshly ground black pepper

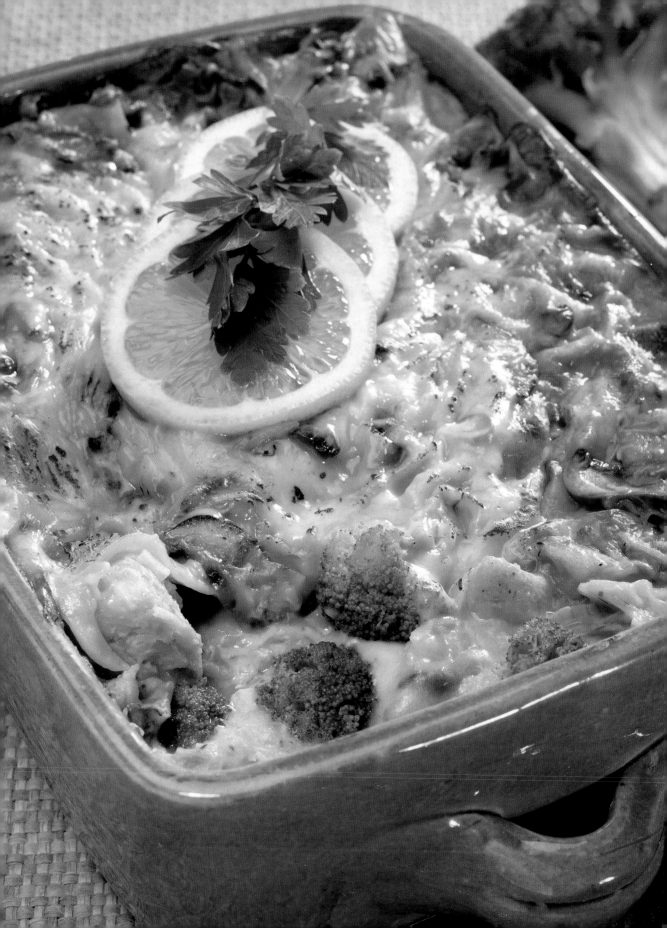

Hot pan smoked salmon

Pan smoking is a variation of barbecuing with the food being totally encased in the cooking smoke. The food is cooked in a smoker over wood chippings, which adds flavour directly to the food.

1 Preheat the oven to 200C, 400F, Gas Mark 6.
2 Prepare the salmon by removing any bones and cut away the skin with a sharp knife. Slice each piece in half and season well with salt and freshly ground black pepper.
3 Prepare the smoker and place the salmon pieces onto the wire rack and cover the whole smoker with aluminium foil, standing the smoker over a low heat.
4 Smoke for 8–10 minutes, reducing the heat if the smoke smells strong.
5 Turn off the heat and allow the smoker to stand for 2–3 minutes before removing the foil. Transfer the salmon to a baking tray and squeeze the juice of half the lemon over. Place in the preheated oven for 5–6 minutes to finish cooking.
6 Make the sauce by combining the fromage frais with the capers, vinegar and parsley, adding lots of salt and freshly ground black pepper.
7 Check that the fish is cooked right through to the centre and serve straight from the oven with the accompanying sauce, a selection of vegetables and garnish with the remaining half lemon and fresh dill.

SERVES 4
PER SERVING:
358 KCAL/19.4G FAT
PREPARATION TIME:
5 MINUTES
COOKING TIME:
25 MINUTES

4 × 175g (4 × 6oz) pieces
  fresh salmon fillet
1 lemon
300g (10oz) virtually fat
  free fromage frais
2 tablespoons capers,
  chopped
2 teaspoons white wine
  vinegar
1 tablespoon chopped
  fresh parsley
salt and freshly ground
  black pepper
dill sprigs to garnish

Hot pan smoking

This unusual method of cooking only lends itself to certain types of food such as salmon and poultry. Smokers can be purchased in good kitchen shops, but a cheaper alternative is to make your own.

All you need are 4 main items: a large turkey-style roasting tin, a small wire rack to fit inside, some hard wood oak chips (sold alongside barbecue fuel) and aluminium foil.

Simply scatter a few oak chips in the bottom of the tin. Place the rack on top, leaving a gap between the wood chips and the bottom of the rack. The food is then placed on top of the rack and the aluminium foil covers everything. Place the tin directly on the cooker hob and smoke away.

It is very important that you keep the heat as low as possible, since if too much smoke is generated it can lead to the food being ruined with a dark brown film tasting sour and bitter.

Vegetables and side dishes

Fresh vegetables are unlimited, so do make sure you offer a wide selection, taking into account flavours, colours and textures. Here we have included a few more unusual choices to serve alongside more conventional basics.

Mushrooms à la Grecque

Lemon and mushrooms make a wonderful combination and the perfect accompaniment to any fish dishes. Serve hot as a vegetable side dish or cold as a salad. Add a few fresh wild mushrooms for added flavour and colour.

1 In a non-stick pan dry-fry the shallot until soft. Wipe the mushrooms with a damp cloth, add to the pan and cook for 1–2 minutes.
2 Add the remaining ingredients except the chopped parsley and bring to the boil. Cover with a lid and remove the pan from the heat. Allow to cool.
3 Before serving, sprinkle with chopped parsley.

SERVES 6
PER SERVING:
23 KCAL/0.7G FAT
PREPARATION TIME:
5 MINUTES
COOKING TIME:
10 MINUTES

1kg (2lb) small chestnut
   mushrooms
2 long shallots, finely chopped
juice of 2 lemons
2 bay leaves
12 peppercorns
1 teaspoon coriander seed
pinch of sea salt
2 tablespoons herb vinegar
1 tablespoon fresh apple juice
1 tablespoon chopped fresh
   parsley

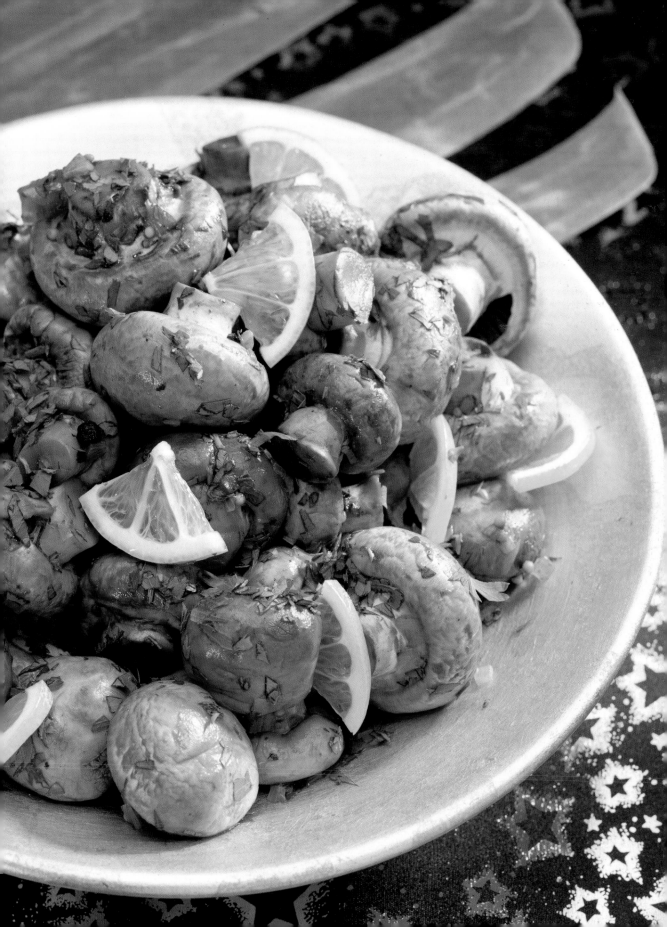

Refried beans

Refried beans are usually a no-no when it comes to low-fat eating, as the main ingredient is half a block of lard to cook everything in. Try them this way and celebrate the absence of unwanted fat.

1 Preheat a non-stick pan until very hot. Drain the kidney beans and rinse well under a running cold tap. Add the beans to the pan and cook over a high heat for 2–3 minutes.
2 Add the garlic and onions and continue to cook for a further 2 minutes. Add the stock and simmer until almost reduced, slightly mashing the beans with the back of a wooden spoon.
3 Fold in the parsley and lettuce and spoon into a serving dish.
4 Garnish with fromage frais and fresh mint.

SERVES 4
PER SERVING:
182 KCAL/6.5G FAT
PREPARATION TIME:
10 MINUTES
COOKING TIME:
25 MINUTES

2 × 400g (2 × 14oz) cans red
   kidney beans
2 garlic cloves, crushed
1 small red onion, finely sliced
8 spring onions, finely chopped
150ml (¼ pint) vegetable stock
1 tablespoon chopped fresh flat
   leaf parsley
6 leaves Romaine lettuce, finely
   shredded
2 tablespoons virtually fat free
   fromage frais to garnish
2–3 sprigs fresh mint to garnish

Sweet red pepper salsa

SERVES 4
PER SERVING:
61 KCAL/0.6G FAT
PREPARATION TIME:
10 MINUTES
COOKING TIME:
30 MINUTES

2 red peppers

1 red onion, finely chopped

4 ripe tomatoes, skinned, seeded
and chopped

zest and juice of 1 lime

1 tablespoon chopped fresh
coriander

1 teaspoon clear honey

salt and freshly ground black
pepper

This salsa can be used as an accompaniment to many dishes. Try it spooned over grilled fish and meat or as a sandwich filler.

1 Cut the peppers in half and remove the seeds. Place skin-side up under a preheated hot grill and leave until black and blistered. Place immediately in a plastic food bag and tie to make airtight. Leave until cold, then carefully peel away the skin under a cold running tap.
2 Dice the peppers and combine with the other ingredients. Season to taste.

Sweet and sour Chinese cabbage

Adding a little sugar to vegetables as they dry-fry helps them to caramelise much quicker, resulting in a much sweeter flavoursome dish.

1 Preheat a non-stick deep wok.
2 Remove 2–3 outer leaves from the cabbage and reserve. Finely shred the inner part of the cabbage. Season well with salt and black pepper.
3 Dry-fry the carrots and cabbage with the sugar over a high heat for 1–2 minutes until they start to caramelise. Pour the tomatoes, soy sauce and vinegar on top and mix well until heated through.
4 Pile into a warmed serving dish, lined with the reserved outer cabbage leaves.

SERVES 4
PER SERVING:
70 KCAL/0.4G FAT
PREPARATION TIME:
10 MINUTES
COOKING TIME:
8 MINUTES

1 Chinese cabbage
2 large carrots, coarsely grated
1 tablespoon soft brown sugar
1 × 400g (14oz) can chopped tomatoes
2 tablespoons light soy sauce
2 tablespoons white wine vinegar
salt and freshly ground black pepper

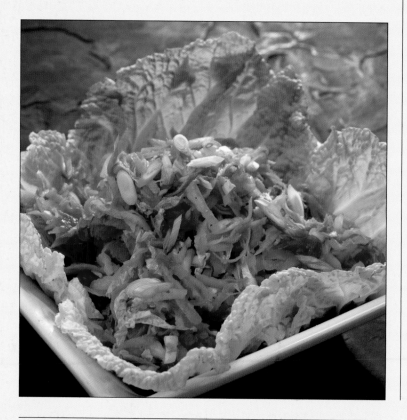

Top right: *Papaya, beansprout and hot banana salad*

Right: *Honey roast corn on the cob*

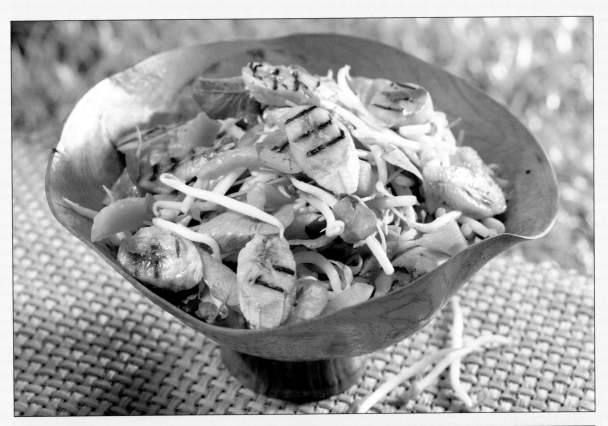

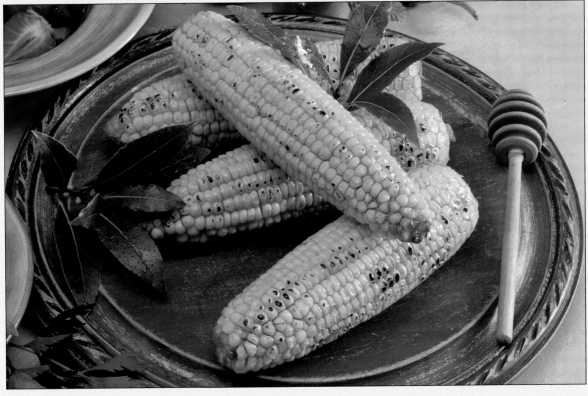

Papaya, beansprout and hot banana salad

Fresh ingredients form an essential part of this recipe. Tired beansprouts and over-ripe papaya will result in a wet, unappetising disaster. Banana takes on a different taste when cooked, so do give it a try and if you can get the cooking variety of plantain this is even better.

1 Peel the papaya, then cut in half and remove the seeds and discard. Cut the flesh into thin strips and place in a large bowl.
2 Wash, drain and pick over the watercress. Add just the tender tops to the bowl, saving the stalks for soup or stock. Add the beansprouts, spring onions and chilli and toss gently to combine the ingredients.
3 Preheat a non-stick frying pan. Peel the bananas and slice on the diagonal to give long slices. Add to the pan and fry quickly for 2–3 minutes on each side so that they are lightly coloured but still firm.
4 Transfer the salad to a serving bowl and arrange the cooked banana on top.
5 Place all the dressing ingredients in a container with a tight-fitting lid – a jam jar is ideal. Shake well until combined, then drizzle over the finished salad. Serve straight away.

See photograph on page 191.

SERVES 4
PER SERVING:
128 KCAL/0.7G FAT
PREPARATION TIME:
15 MINUTES
COOKING TIME:
8 MINUTES

2 ripe papaya
1 small bunch watercress
225g (8oz) fresh beansprouts
6 spring onions, finely chopped
1 small red chilli, finely chopped
2 small green bananas

for the dressing
150ml (1/4 pint) orange juice
3 tablespoons blackberry or raspberry fruit vinegar
1 teaspoon mild Dijon mustard
1 teaspoon clear honey
2 tablespoons finely chopped coriander
salt and freshly ground black pepper to taste

Honey roast corn on the cob

SERVES 4
PER SERVING:
172 KCAL/2.15G FAT
PREPARATION TIME:
10 MINUTES
COOKING TIME:
35 MINUTES

4 large corn on the cob
1 vegetable stock cube
1 teaspoon ground cumin
2 tablespoons runny honey
salt and freshly ground black
    pepper
a few chopped fresh chives to
    garnish

Corn on the cob tends to go hand in hand with lashings of high-fat butter. Enjoy them just as much with a sticky coating of sweet honey.

1 Preheat the oven to 200C, 400F, Gas Mark 6.
2 Remove the outer husk and silky threads from the cobs of corn and trim the ends with a sharp knife.
3 In a large saucepan dissolve the stock cube in approximately 1.2 litres (2 pints) water. Add the cumin and bring to the boil.
4 Carefully add the corn to the pan and top up with boiling water from a kettle so that the corn is completely covered. Simmer gently for 10–12 minutes until the kernels are tender when teased out with the point of a knife. Drain through a colander and place in a roasting tray. Drizzle with honey and season with salt and black pepper.
5 Place in the preheated oven for 15–20 minutes until lightly roasted.
6 Serve hot or cold with a sprinkling of chopped fresh chives.

See photograph on page 191.

Baby carrots and broad beans in a lemon sauce

Broad beans can dry out very quickly. Try adding a rich creamy lemon sauce – it can really make all the difference. This sauce can also be used alongside other vegetables as well as fish and meat dishes.

1 Top and tail the carrots and place in a large saucepan. Cover with water and boil with a pinch of salt for 10–12 minutes.

2 Add the broad beans, bring back to the boil and simmer gently until the beans are cooked.

3 In a separate pan heat the milk with the bay leaves and stock cube to near boiling. Slake the cornflour with a little cold water and whisk into the hot milk. Keep stirring as the sauce thickens. Add the mustard and lemon zest and juice and season well with salt and black pepper.

4 Drain the vegetables into a serving dish, spoon the sauce over and sprinkle with chopped fresh parsley.

SERVES 4
PER SERVING:
110 KCAL / 1.6G FAT
PREPARATION TIME:
20 MINUTES
COOKING TIME:
20 MINUTES

225g (8oz) young baby carrots, scraped
225g (8oz) shelled baby broad beans
300ml (½ pint) skimmed milk
2 bay leaves
1 vegetable stock cube
4 teaspoons cornflour
2 teaspoons Dijon mustard
zest and juice of 1 lemon
salt and freshly ground black pepper
1 tablespoon chopped fresh parsley to garnish

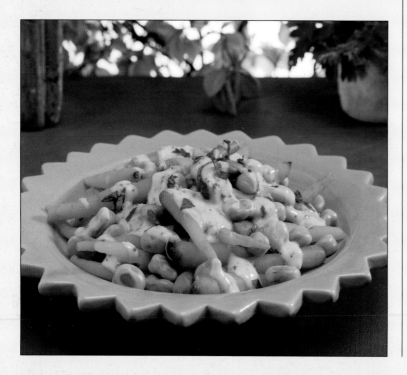

Garlic and herb roasted new potatoes

SERVES 4
PER SERVING:
85 KCAL/0.4G FAT
PREPARATION TIME:
15 MINUTES
COOKING TIME:
45 MINUTES

450g (1lb) new potatoes
2 garlic cloves, finely chopped
2–3 sprigs fresh rosemary
2–3 sprigs fresh thyme
2 tablespoons light soy sauce
chopped fresh thyme or
    coriander to garnish

This is a great way of dressing up leftover cooked potatoes. A good tip is to roast off a large quantity and portion them for the freezer. Cook straight from frozen in a hot oven.

1 Preheat the oven to 200C, 400F, Gas Mark 6.
2 Cook the potatoes in boiling salted water. Drain and place in a non-stick roasting tin.
3 Sprinkle with the garlic and herbs, pulling the leaves away from the stems.
4 Drizzle with soy sauce and toss the potatoes, coating them with the mixture.
5 Place in the preheated oven and roast for 35–45 minutes, shaking the pan occasionally to prevent sticking.
6 Transfer to a serving bowl and garnish with chopped fresh thyme or coriander.

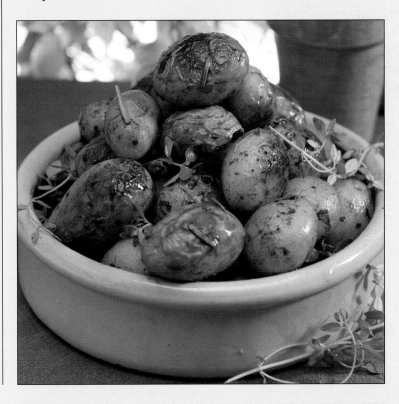

Vegetable brunoise

A colourful combination of vegetables. Cutting them small reduces the cooking time considerably. Leftover vegetables can be mixed with a little low-fat fromage frais for a creamy vegetable salad, the perfect accompaniment to cold meats.

1 Prepare all the vegetables by cutting each one into regular small dice.
2 Place the carrots, squash and swede into a saucepan and cover with water, add the stock cube and bring to the boil. Simmer for 2–3 minutes, then add the remaining vegetables. Simmer until tender, then drain.
3 Just before serving, garnish with sprigs of fresh mint.

SERVES 4
PER SERVING:
70 KCAL/0.7G FAT
PREPARATION TIME:
15 MINUTES
COOKING TIME:
10 MINUTES

4 medium sized carrots, peeled
1/2 butternut squash, peeled
1 small swede, peeled
1 vegetable stock cube
2 small sweet potatoes, peeled
2 small courgettes
2–3 spring onions, chopped
fresh mint to garnish

Potatoes marquise

SERVES 4
PER SERVING:
169 KCAL/0.8G FAT
PREPARATION TIME:
30 MINUTES
COOKING TIME:
25 MINUTES

675g (1 1/2 lb) potatoes, peeled
    and chopped

2 tablespoons skimmed milk

1 tablespoon virtually fat free
    fromage frais

1 medium onion, finely chopped

1 garlic clove, crushed

6 tomatoes, skinned, seeded and
    chopped

salt and freshly ground black
    pepper

2 tablespoons chopped fresh
    chives to garnish

1 Preheat the oven to 200C, 400F, Gas Mark 6.
2 Boil the potatoes in salted water until cooked, drain well and mash with a potato masher, adding the skimmed milk and fromage frais until lump free.
3 Dry-fry the onion and garlic in a preheated non-stick pan until it starts to colour. Add the tomatoes and remove from the heat.
4 Take a large piping bag with a star nozzle and fill with the potato mixture. On a non-stick baking tray pipe round discs of potato, 8cm (4in) in diameter, then pipe a second layer on top of each disc but only around the perimeter, leaving a void in the centre. Spoon the tomato mixture into the centre.
5 Bake in the preheated oven for 20–25 minutes until brown and crispy.
6 Serve hot, sprinkled with chives.

See photograph on page 198.

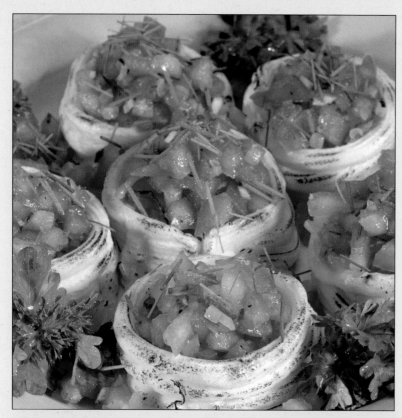

Left: *Potatoes marquise*

Below: *Baked creamed cauliflower*

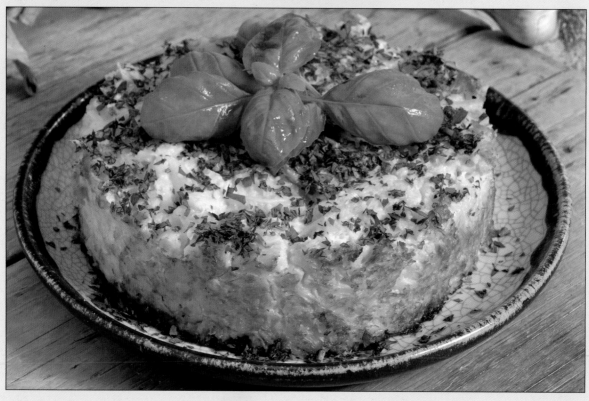

Braised fennel

SERVES 4
PER SERVING:
21 KCAL/0.3G FAT
PREPARATION TIME:
10 MINUTES
COOKING TIME:
50 MINUTES

8 small heads fennel

2 garlic cloves, crushed

1 teaspoon chopped fresh
thyme

3–4 juniper berries, crushed

2 teaspoons vegetable bouillon
stock powder

salt and freshly ground black
pepper

4 ripe tomatoes, skinned, seeded
and diced to garnish

chopped fresh chives to garnish

*Fennel is an interesting vegetable with a strong anise flavour.
Florence fennel is small and sweet and can be eaten both raw in
salads and cooked as a vegetable. It is also a great addition to
vegetable soups.*

1 Trim away the root from the bottom of the fennel bulbs. Split
each bulb down the centre with a sharp knife, then cut into
small wedges.

2 Preheat a non-stick frying pan until hot, add the fennel and
cook quickly over a high heat for 5–6 minutes until they start
to colour. Add the garlic and continue cooking for 1–2 minutes.

3 Sprinkle the thyme, juniper and stock powder over the fennel,
then pour 300ml (½ pint) boiling water into the pan. Season
with black pepper, cover with a lid and braise gently for 10–15
minutes until tender.

4 Pour into a serving dish and sprinkle with the diced tomato and
chopped fresh chives.

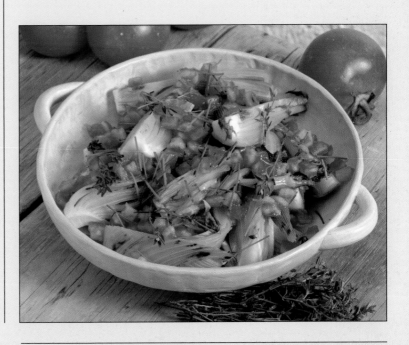

Baked creamed cauliflower

The mustard in this recipe gives the cauliflower a real lift. This vegetable accompaniment will be quite safe left in a low oven until ready to serve. Try adding fresh basil or even a little blue cheese to the mixture.

1 Preheat the oven to 200C, 400F, Gas Mark 6.
2 Remove the outer leaves from the cauliflower and break the vegetable into florets. Cook in a pan of boiling salted water until tender, then drain well.
3 In a small saucepan heat the milk with the stock and garlic until boiling. Slake the cornflour with a little cold milk and whisk into the hot milk. Simmer gently for 1–2 minutes, stirring well as the sauce thickens.
4 Remove the sauce from the heat and beat in the mustard and egg, seasoning well with salt and black pepper.
5 Place the drained cauliflower into a large bowl and break up slightly with a fork. Add the sauce and mix well. Pour into a small, round, non-stick cake tin and smooth the top with the back of a fork.
6 Place in the oven and bake for 30 minutes.
7 To serve, run a knife around the inside edge of the tin, place a serving plate on top, invert and turn out on to the plate. Sprinkle with parsley and serve.

See photograph on page 198.

SERVES 4
PER SERVING:
117 KCAL/3.2G FAT
PREPARATION TIME:
10 MINUTES
COOKING TIME:
50 MINUTES

1 medium cauliflower
300ml (½ pint) skimmed milk
1 teaspoon vegetable bouillon
    stock powder
1 garlic clove, crushed
1 tablespoon cornflour
1 tablespoon Dijon mustard
1 egg, beaten
salt and freshly ground black
    pepper
2 tablespoons chopped fresh
    parsley to garnish

Puddings

For chocolate lovers and the rest of us, here are some more tempting recipes that, without doubt, taste delicious and luxurious, even though the fat and calories have been reduced.

Some of the more substantial recipes are designed to follow a light meal, so calculate accordingly and indulge without guilt.

Banana split with hot chocolate sauce

A dessert to die for! Although low in fat, this dessert makes up for it in calories so make sure you compensate your main meals accordingly.

1 In a small saucepan heat the cocoa powder with the milk, whisking continuously.
2 Slake the cornflour with a little cold milk and whisk into the milk. Simmer for 1 minute as the sauce thickens, then add sugar to taste. Keep warm over a low heat.
3 Peel the bananas, slice in half lengthways and place in a serving dish. Sprinkle with the lemon juice to prevent them turning brown.
4 Divide the raspberries between the 4 dishes. Place 2 scoops of iced dessert on top of the raspberries then pour the chocolate sauce over.
5 Serve straight away.

SERVES 4
PER SERVING:
199 KCAL / 4.4G FAT
PREPARATION TIME:
10 MINUTES
COOKING TIME:
20 MINUTES

1 tablespoon Valrhona cocoa powder
300ml ($\frac{1}{2}$ pint) semi–skimmed milk
2 teaspoons cornflour
1 tablespoon caster sugar
4 small ripe bananas
2 tablespoons lemon juice
225g (8oz) fresh raspberries
8 scoops Wall's 'Too Good To Be True' iced dessert

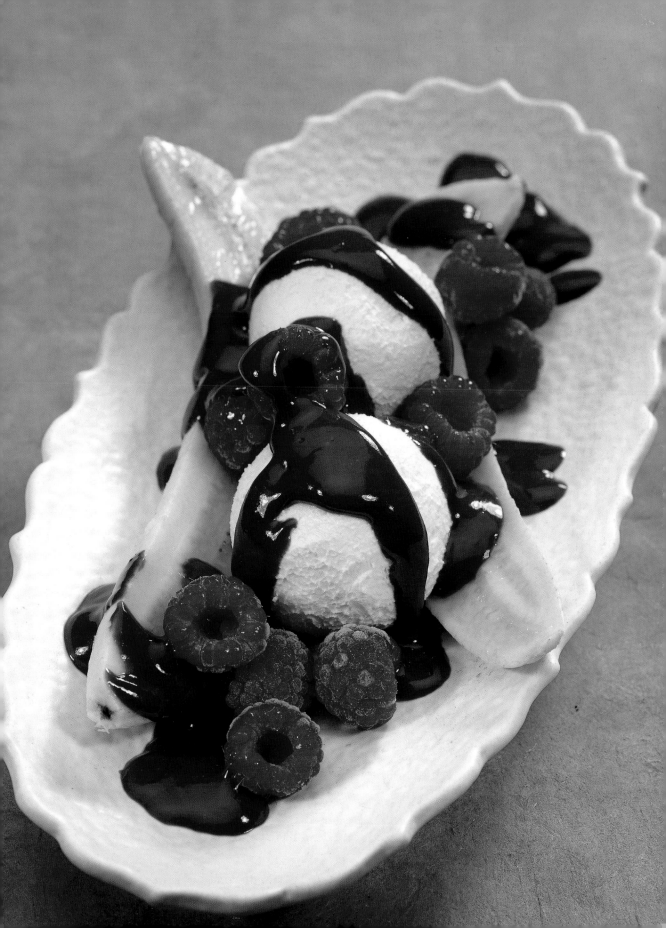

Summer berry gratin

Any combination of fruit may be used in this recipe. Firm fruits such as blueberries or peaches are cooked in a little wine for added flavour. The egg white adds bulk and a lighter texture.

1 Place the blueberries in a small saucepan and add the wine and sugar. Cook gently over a low heat until the fruit starts to pop.
2 Turn off the heat, add the raspberries and strawberries and mix well. Spoon into 4 gratin or shallow dishes and chill.
3 When the fruit is chilled, preheat the grill until it is very hot.
4 Just before you are ready to serve, whisk the egg whites to stiff peaks and fold into the yogurt. Spread the yogurt over the fruit, covering the fruit completely. Sprinkle with demerara sugar and immediately place under the grill until the sugar caramelises.
5 Serve immediately.

SERVES 4
PER SERVING:
225 KCAL/1.1G FAT
PREPARATION TIME:
10 MINUTES
COOKING TIME:
15 MINUTES

175g (6oz) blueberries
½ wine glass white wine
2 tablespoons caster sugar
175g (6oz) raspberries
175g (6oz) strawberries, hulled
   and sliced
2 egg whites
600g (1lb 5oz) Total 0% fat
   Greek yogurt
4 tablespoons demerara sugar

Pineapple crush

SERVES 6
PER SERVING:
180 KCAL/2.6G FAT
PREPARATION TIME:
20 MINUTES
COOKING TIME:
5 MINUTES

1 large pineapple
225g (8oz) low-fat sponge
   fingers
2 tablespoons dry sherry
2 egg whites
300ml (½ pint) Total 0% Greek
   yogurt
icing sugar

1 Prepare the pineapple by slicing off the top and bottom with a sharp knife. Remove the outer skin, slicing down the fruit. Cut the fruit lengthways into quarters and remove the central core.

2 Place the sponge fingers into a food processor and reduce to fine crumbs, pour into a bowl, sprinkle with the sherry and set aside.

3 Roughly chop the pineapple and add to the food processor. Using the pulse motion, reduce the flesh to a chunky purée.

4 Whisk the egg whites until stiff, then gradually fold in the yogurt and icing sugar.

5 Assemble the dessert in a glass dish or in individual sundae glasses in layers, first with sponge finger crumbs sprinkled with sherry, then pineapple and finally the yogurt mixture. Repeat, dusting the top with crumbs.

6 Refrigerate until ready to serve.

See photograph on page 206.

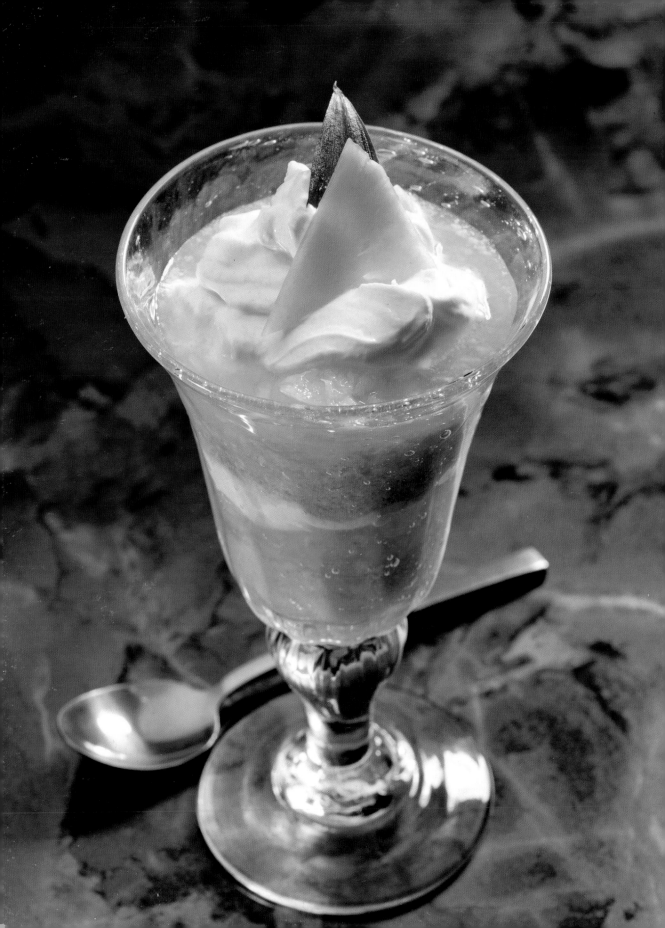

Apricot and almond syllabub

SERVES 1
PER SERVING:
174 KCAL / 1.4G FAT
PREPARATION TIME:
10 MINUTES
COOKING TIME:
15 MINUTES

25g (1oz) dried apricots
zest and juice of 1 lime
4–5 tablespoons low-fat Greek
   yogurt
2 teaspoons Amaretto liqueur
1 egg white

1 Place the apricots and lime into a small saucepan and cover with water. Bring to the boil and simmer until soft and virtually all the water has evaporated. Using a fork, mash the apricots until smooth.
2 Beat the yogurt into the apricot mixture, add the liqueur and sweeten to taste with a little sugar. Whisk the egg white to stiff peaks and gently fold into the mixture.
3 Spoon into a glass and chill until required.

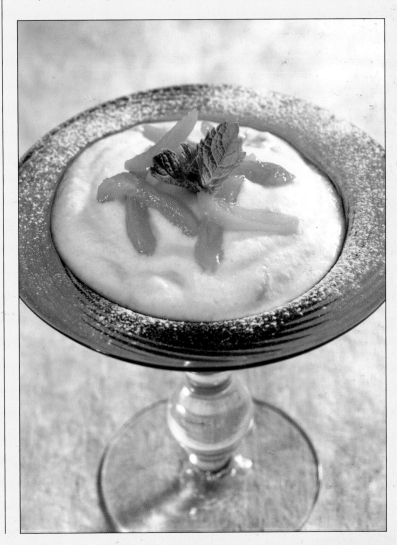

Left: *Pineapple crush*

Valrhona chocolate mousse

Valrhona cocoa powder is made using a high quantity of cocoa solids, thus giving a much stronger fuller chocolate flavour. To create a completely decadent dessert, grate a little white chocolate from a 10g Nestle's Milky Bar to give a touch of luxury on top.

1 Heat the milk and cocoa powder in a small saucepan. Slake the cornflour with a little cold water and whisk into the hot milk, along with the sugar. Simmer until the sauce thickens, remove from the heat, pour into a mixing bowl and allow to cool.

2 Soak the gelatine in cold water for 2–3 minutes until it becomes soft. Place it in a bowl and heat it either over a pan of boiling water or in a microwave for 1 minute until liquid. Add to the chocolate sauce, mixing in well, along with the fromage frais.

3 Whisk the egg whites until stiff and fold into the mixture. Spoon into individual glasses or place in a glass bowl.

4 Decorate with grated white chocolate, redcurrants and mint leaves.

SERVES 6
PER SERVING:
188 KCAL / 1.4G FAT
PREPARATION TIME:
5 MINUTES
COOKING TIME:
15 MINUTES

300ml (½ pint) semi-skimmed milk
2 tablespoons Valrhona cocoa powder
2 tablespoons cornflour
115g (4oz) caster sugar
6 sheets leaf gelatine
450g (16oz) virtually fat free Normandy fromage frais
3 egg whites
1 × 10g Milky Bar
a few redcurrants to decorate
a few mint leaves to decorate

Chocolate marble puddings

SERVES 4
PER SERVING:
302 KCAL/2.8G FAT
PREPARATION TIME:
5 MINUTES
COOKING TIME:
30 MINUTES

115g (4oz) Quark (low-fat cheese)

115g (4oz) caster sugar

1 egg yolk

2 egg whites

150g (5oz) plain flour

2 teaspoons baking powder

3 tablespoons orange juice

1 tablespoon Valrhona cocoa powder

Create a stir with these stunning chocolate puddings. For a fruitier pudding add 2–3 teaspoons of marmalade to the bottom of each ramekin.

1 Preheat the oven to 180C, 350F, Gas Mark 4. Lightly grease 4 × 115g (4 × 4oz) ramekin dishes.
2 In a mixing bowl beat together the Quark, sugar and egg yolk until smooth. Beat in the flour and baking powder.
3 In a clean bowl whisk the egg whites until stiff and fold into the mixture.
4 In a small bowl gradually mix the orange juice into the cocoa powder to form a smooth paste. Pour the cocoa over the sponge mixture and stir to create a marbled effect.
5 Spoon into prepared dishes and bake in the centre of the preheated oven for 15–20 minutes until well risen and firm to the touch.
6 Serve hot with low-fat yogurt or fromage frais.

Caramel coffee pears with vanilla sauce

Choose firm pears without bruising, as the discoloration caused by bruising will show once peeled. The vanilla sauce can be made in advance and stored with a disc of parchment paper on the top to avoid a skin forming.

1 Peel the pears and cut in half lengthways. Scoop out the core with a spoon and rub the surface of the pears with the lemon juice. Place the pears in a large bowl and sprinkle the sugar over to coat.

2 Preheat a non-stick saucepan. Add the pears, placing them face down in the pan. Cook gently until the sugar starts to caramelise, then add the coffee and continue cooking until the pears soften.

3 In the meantime, make the sauce by heating the milk in a saucepan. Split the vanilla pod lengthways and scrape the blade of the knife along the inside edges of the pod to remove the seeds. Add these to the milk along with the pod.

4 Slake the cornflour with a little cold water and whisk into the hot milk. Simmer gently to allow the sauce to thicken.

5 Arrange the pears in a serving dish and pour the sauce around.

SERVES 4
PER SERVING:
255 KCAL / 1.4G FAT
PREPARATION TIME:
5 MINUTES
COOKING TIME:
20 MINUTES

4 large firm pears
2 tablespoons lemon juice
115g (4oz) caster sugar
50ml (2fl oz) coffee
300ml (½ pint) semi-skimmed milk
1 vanilla pod
2 teaspoons cornflour
sugar to taste

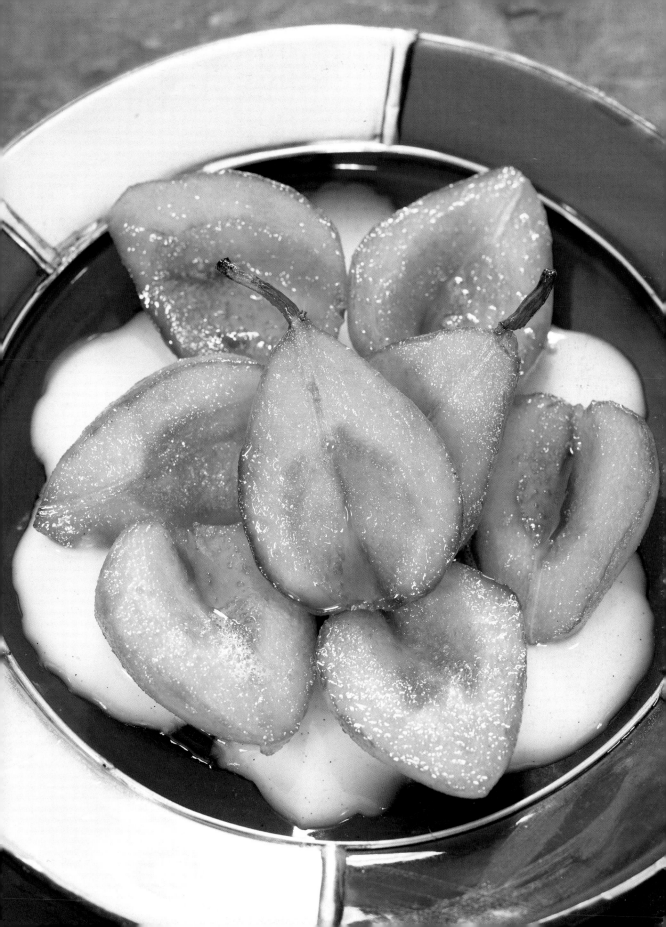

Mexican candy

Indulge in this crisp, orange-flavoured candy. Delicious dipped in hot strong coffee.

1 Lightly grease a 20cm (8in) square non-stick tin.
2 Scatter the raisins over the base of the prepared tin.
3 Heat the sugar with the water over a low heat in a heavy bottom saucepan until it starts to melt into a liquid. Using a wooden spoon, draw the mixture from the outside into the middle of the pan. When the sugar has caramelised, turned a golden brown colour and has completely dissolved, carefully pour over the raisins, standing well back in case the caramel spits.
4 Using a fine grater, grate the orange zest over. Allow to cool and set.
5 Cut or break into pieces and serve.

MAKES 8 PIECES
PER PIECE 188 KCAL/0.03G FAT
PREPARATION TIME: 5 MINUTES
COOKING TIME: 30 MINUTES

1 tablespoon raisins
350g (12oz) caster sugar
4 tablespoons water
fine zest of 1 orange

Orange velvet cream

SERVES 4
PER SERVING:
188 KCAL/0.9G FAT
PREPARATION TIME:
20 MINUTES
COOKING TIME:
15 MINUTES

4 oranges
1 tablespoon caster sugar
2 heaped tablespoons custard
   powder
250ml (8fl oz) skimmed milk
300g (11oz) low-fat Greek
   yogurt
2 egg whites
orange segments and mint
   leaves to decorate

1 Zest the oranges on a fine grater into a small bowl. Squeeze the juice from 2 of the oranges into the bowl.
2 In a separate bowl mix together the sugar and custard powder with a little cold milk to form a smooth paste.
3 Heat the remaining milk in a saucepan until boiling, pour onto the custard powder and whisk well. Return to the pan and cook until the mixture starts to thicken, then stir in the orange zest and juice. Remove from the heat, cover with food wrap and allow to cool.
4 Once cold, beat the yogurt into the custard mixture and sweeten to taste with a little sugar.
5 Whisk the egg whites to stiff peaks and gently fold into the mixture. Spoon into individual glasses or a large serving bowl and decorate with orange segments and mint.

Black cherry clafoutis

Clafoutis is a batter pudding baked with fruit. The original, from the Limousin province of France, was made with freshly gathered black cherries. If you find them too fiddly to stone, substitute with drained canned cherries.

1 Preheat the oven to 200C, 400F, Gas Mark 6.
2 De-stalk and stone the cherries and place in the bottom of a lightly greased shallow ovenproof dish. Drizzle with the cherry liqueur.
3 In a mixing bowl beat together the eggs and sugar until thick and creamy. Gradually blend in the flour to a smooth paste, adding a little milk if necessary.
4 Heat the milk with the vanilla in a small saucepan until near boiling. Slowly pour the milk onto the batter, stirring continuously. Pour the batter over the cherries.
5 Bake in the preheated oven for 25–30 minutes until set.
6 Serve warm with low-fat fromage frais.

SERVES 4
PER SERVING:
192 KCAL/3.2G FAT
PREPARATION TIME:
20 MINUTES
COOKING TIME:
40 MINUTES

450g (1lb) black cherries
2 tablespoons cherry liqueur
2 eggs
3 1/2 tablespoons caster sugar
1 level tablespoon plain flour
300ml (1/2 pint) skimmed milk
1 teaspoon vanilla extract

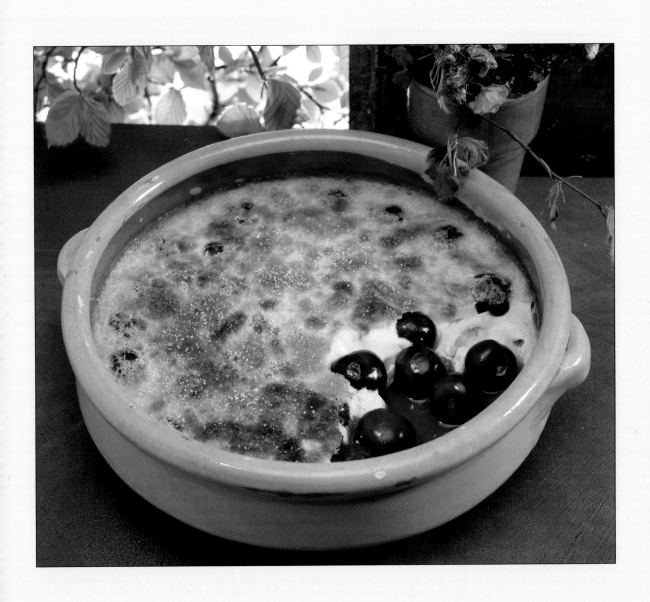

Blackberry and apple crisp

This is a lighter version of a traditional high-fat fruit crumble. While high in calories, this is a great low-fat dessert treat to have after a low-calorie main course. Vary the filling by using different combinations of seasonal fruits. Slicing apples into salted water prevents them from discolouring. Remember to rinse them well in fresh water before using to remove the salt.

1 Preheat the oven to 200C, 400F, Gas Mark 6.
2 Spread the breadcrumbs on a baking sheet and sprinkle with the brown sugar. Bake in the oven for 20 minutes, stirring occasionally until the sugar caramelises and the crumbs are toasted. Cool and break down with a fork or food processor and place in a mixing bowl.
3 Peel, core and slice the apples into a bowl of water containing the salt. Rinse well and place in the bottom of an ovenproof dish. Scatter the blackberries over the top and sprinkle with the caster sugar. Pour the orange juice over.
4 Mix the orange zest and cinnamon into the breadcrumbs and scatter evenly over the fruit.
5 Bake in the oven for 25–30 minutes until the fruit is cooked through and the topping browned.
6 Serve warm with low-fat fromage frais.

SERVES 6
PER SERVING:
264 KCAL/0.8G FAT
PREPARATION TIME:
10 MINUTES
COOKING TIME:
30 MINUTES

225g (8oz) fresh brown
    breadcrumbs
115g (4oz) soft brown sugar
450g (1lb) cooking apples
1 tablespoon salt
225g (8oz) blackberries
2 tablespoons caster sugar
zest and juice of 1 orange
1 teaspoon ground cinnamon

Apple tart

A cheat's tart using fat-free sponge as a base to this fruity dessert. The apples need to be sliced into either salted water or lemon juice to prevent them turning brown. Add a little spice if you wish in the form of ground cinnamon or ground cloves.

SERVES 6
PER SERVING:
249 KCAL/2.5G FAT
PREPARATION TIME:
20 MINUTES
COOKING TIME:
60 MINUTES

2 eggs
75g (3oz) golden caster sugar
75g (3oz) self-raising flour, sifted
1 teaspoon vanilla essence
1kg (2lb) cooking apples
1–2 tablespoons golden caster sugar
2 red eating apples
1 tablespoon lemon juice
1 tablespoon Calvados brandy
salt
apricot jam to glaze

1 Preheat the oven to 180C, 350F, Gas Mark 4. Grease a 20cm (8in) non-stick flan case with a little vegetable oil, then dust with caster sugar.

2 To make the sponge base, whisk together the eggs and sugar for several minutes until thick and pale in consistency. Using a metal spoon, fold in the sifted flour then the vanilla. Pour into the prepared tin and level off with a knife. Bake in the oven for 20 minutes until golden brown.

3 Allow the sponge to cool, then, using a serrated knife, cut away a 1cm ($\frac{1}{2}$in) layer of sponge from the centre of the flan case. Using a metal spoon, scrape away the crumbs to leave a smooth surface.

4 Peel, core and slice the cooking apples into a bowl of salted water. Rinse the apples well in fresh water then cook in a non-stick pan over a low heat for 15–20 minutes until soft.

5 Stir in the sugar to sweeten to taste, drain the apples through a metal sieve to remove any excess liquid then spoon into the sponge case.

6 Core the eating apples and cut in half. Thinly slice into a bowl containing the lemon juice. Cook the apple slices in the bottom of a non-stick frying pan until soft then arrange on the top of the flan.

7 Heat the Calvados with a little apricot jam in a small saucepan and brush over the top to glaze the apples.

8 Serve cold with virtually fat free fromage frais or Total 0% fat Greek yogurt.

See photograph on page 218.

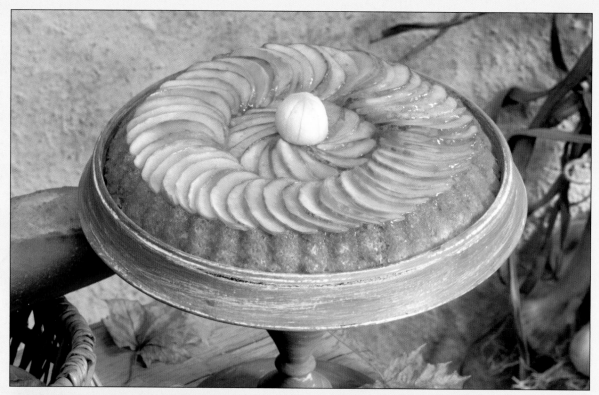

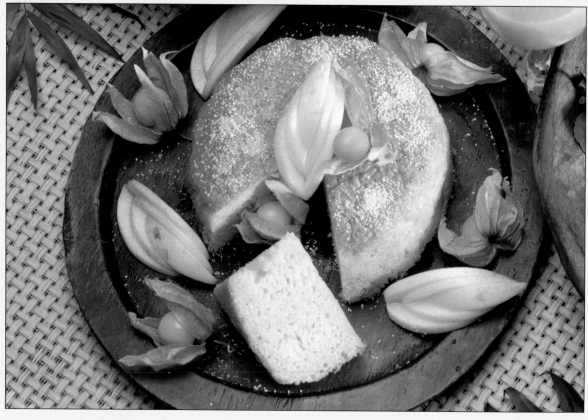

Pear and lemon polenta cake

SERVES 4
PER SERVING:
316 KCAL/5.2G FAT
PREPARATION TIME:
10 MINUTES
COOKING TIME:
40 MINUTES

175g (6oz) canned pears in
    natural juice, drained
115g (4oz) caster sugar
75g (3oz) plain flour
50g (2oz) fine polenta
3 eggs, beaten
2 lemons
1 teaspoon baking powder

Polenta is a versatile flour produced from ground maize or corn, hence the rich golden colour of this nutty flavoured cake.

1 Preheat the oven to 180C, 350F, Gas Mark 4. Prepare a 15cm (6in) round cake tin by lightly greasing with a little margarine, then line with greaseproof paper.
2 Drain the pears well, place in a large mixing bowl and mash down to a pulp with a large fork.
3 Beat in the sugar, using a wooden spoon, then add the flour, polenta and eggs a little at a time.
4 Using a fine grater, add the zest of both lemons plus the juice of one.
5 Finally, beat in the baking powder and pour into the prepared tin.
6 Bake in the oven for 40 minutes until a skewer inserted comes out clean.
7 Allow to cool then drizzle with the lemon juice from the remaining lemon.
8 Slice and serve with low-fat fromage frais and additional pears.

Top left: *Apple tart*

Left: *Pear and lemon polenta cake*

Sauces and dressings

Low-fat sauces are very easy to make. Adding fresh herbs or other ingredients can change a sauce completely, which can make all the difference to a meal. Included in this section are basil pesto and other, more common, high-fat accompaniments – all made the low-fat way.

Fat-free mayonnaise

MAKES 220ML (7 1/2 FL OZ)
PER TABLESPOON:
9 KCAL/0.02G FAT

175g (6oz) virtually fat free
fromage frais
2 tablespoons cider vinegar
1 tablespoon lemon juice
1/4 teaspoon ground turmeric
2 teaspoons sugar
salt and freshly ground black
pepper

Real mayonnaise contains egg yolks and oil, two very high-fat ingredients. We have managed to develop a low-fat dressing that can be substituted in recipes containing mayonnaise. The turmeric adds a rich golden colour to the finished dressing.

1 Combine all the ingredients in a small bowl.
2 Whisk until smooth. Store in the refrigerator and use within 3 days.

Fresh basil yogurt dressing

SERVES 6
PER SERVING:
22 KCAL/0.3G FAT

175g (6oz) low-fat natural
yogurt
1 tablespoon lemon juice
2 tablespoons chopped fresh
basil
1 garlic clove, crushed
1 teaspoon clear honey
salt and freshly ground black
pepper

Basil has a strong and perfumed flavour. Its affinity with tomatoes is longstanding. Spoon this dressing over a simple tomato and red onion salad and leave to marinate for 20 minutes.

1 Combine all the ingredients in a small bowl.
2 Whisk until smooth, season well with salt and pepper. Store in the refrigerator and use within 4 days.

Fresh basil pesto

Basil pesto can be bought in many forms from jars to sachets, however the majority are made with a high percentage of fat. The chestnuts add a little body, but if you prefer they may be left out.

1 Dissolve the stock cube in 150ml (1/4 pint) boiling water.
2 Pluck the basil leaves from the main plant stem and place in a food processor or liquidiser.
3 Add the remaining ingredients and blend until smooth. Season to taste with salt and freshly ground black pepper and scrape out into a bowl.

SERVES 4
PER SERVING:
11 KCAL/0.7G FAT

1 vegetable stock cube
2 good bunches fresh basil
1 garlic clove, crushed
1 tablespoon finely chopped peeled cooked chestnuts
2 teaspoons grated fresh Parmesan cheese
salt and freshly ground black pepper

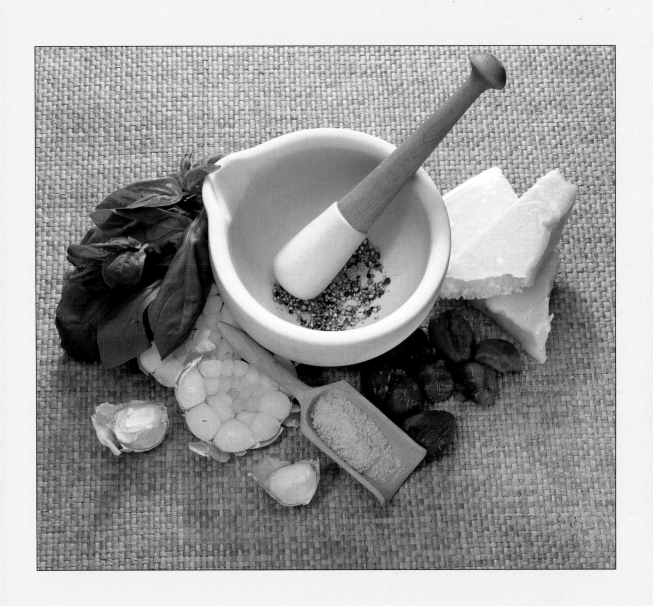

Honey and orange dressing

This dressing can be stored in the refrigerator for one week.

1 Place the orange juice, honey and vinegar in a pan. Add the Dijon mustard and orange rind.
2 Bring to the boil, allow to cool and add the chopped chives and parsley. Season to taste with salt and freshly ground black pepper.

SERVES 6
PER SERVING:
18 KCAL/0G FAT

6 tablespoons orange juice
4 teaspoons thin honey
1 tablespoon white wine
    vinegar
½ teaspoon Dijon wholegrain
    mustard
1 teaspoon grated orange rind
2 teaspoons chopped fresh
    chives and parsley, mixed
salt and freshly ground black
    pepper to taste

Prawn cocktail sauce

1 Mix all the ingredients together.
2 Store in a screw-top jar in the refrigerator until required.

SERVES 1
PER SERVING:
50 KCAL/0.5G FAT

1 tablespoon tomato ketchup
½ tablespoon reduced-oil salad
    dressing
1 tablespoon low-fat natural
    yogurt
black pepper to taste
dash of Tabasco sauce

Yogurt and mint dressing

SERVES 4
PER SERVING:
28 KCAL/0.4G FAT

175g (6oz) low-fat natural
    yogurt
1–2 teaspoons mint sauce
1 tablespoon finely chopped
    fresh parsley
salt and freshly ground black
    pepper to taste

1 Mix all the ingredients together in a container.
2 Store in the refrigerator and use within 2 days.

Balsamic dressing

SERVES 6
PER SERVING:
17 KCAL/0.4G FAT

300ml (½ pint) apple juice
2 tablespoons balsamic vinegar
1 tablespoon mild Dijon
    mustard
pinch of sugar
salt and freshly ground black
    pepper

Balsamic vinegar is a dark sweet vinegar from Modena in Italy. Its rich syrupy consistency makes a delicious fruity dressing.

1 Combine all the ingredients in a small bowl and whisk until smooth.
2 Place in a sealed jar or bottle and use as required. Use within 5 days.

Caesar salad dressing

Sometimes salad dressing can become repetitive, so pep it up with a few extra ingredients.

1 Combine all the ingredients in a bowl, cover and refrigerate for 1 hour to allow the flavours to develop.
2 Serve with grilled fish, meat or roasted vegetables.

SERVES 4
PER SERVING:
25 KCAL/0.9G FAT

4 tablespoons low-fat salad dressing
1 tablespoon fat-free fromage frais
1 garlic clove, crushed
2–3 teaspoons fresh lemon juice
2 teaspoons grated fresh Parmesan cheese
salt and freshly ground black pepper

White sauce

1 Heat all but 50ml (2fl oz) of the milk in a non-stick saucepan, adding the onion, peppercorns, bay leaf and seasoning.
2 Heat gently and cover the pan. Simmer for 5 minutes. Turn off the heat and leave the milk mixture to stand with the lid on for a further 30 minutes or until you are ready to thicken and serve the sauce.
3 Mix the remaining milk with the cornflour and when it's almost time to serve it, strain the milk, add the cornflour mixture and reheat slowly, stirring continuously until it comes to the boil. If it begins to thicken too quickly, remove from the heat and stir very fast to mix well.
4 Cook for 3–4 minutes and serve immediately.

SERVES 4
PER SERVING:
55 KCAL/0.2G FAT

300ml ($\frac{1}{2}$pint) skimmed milk
1 onion, peeled and sliced
6 peppercorns
1 bay leaf
2 teaspoons cornflour
salt and freshly ground black pepper

Chilli barbecue sauce

SERVES 4
PER SERVING:
48 KCAL / 0.2G FAT

1 onion
1 garlic clove
150ml (¼ pint) tomato juice
2 tablespoons Worcestershire
   sauce
1 teaspoon medium hot chilli
   powder or to taste
4 tablespoons white wine
   vinegar
2 tablespoons clear honey
2 tablespoons soy sauce
1 teaspoon French mustard
salt and freshly ground black
   pepper

1 Peel the onion and garlic. Finely chop the onion and crush the garlic. Place in a small pan.
2 Add the remaining ingredients and mix well.
3 Bring slowly to the boil and simmer for 15 minutes or until the onions are soft. Add a little water if necessary to prevent the sauce becoming too thick. Taste and check the seasoning and adjust the consistency with more water at the end of the cooking time. Serve hot.

Mustard sauce

A delicious sauce served with gammon or a good base sauce for lasagne or a pasta bake.

1 Heat the milk and stock cube in a non-stick saucepan until stock cube has dissolved.
2 Mix the cornflour with a little water to a paste, add slowly to the milk, stirring well until it comes to the boil. Cook for 2–3 minutes.
3 Stir in the mustard and parsley. Adjust the consistency with a little water if required. Season to taste.

SERVES 4
PER SERVING:
59 KCAL/1.2G FAT

300ml (½ pint) skimmed milk
1 vegetable stock cube
2 teaspoons cornflour
1½ tablespoons Dijon mustard
1 tablespoon chopped fresh
    parsley (optional)
salt and freshly ground black
    pepper

Parsley sauce

1 Heat all but 50ml (2fl oz) of the milk in a non-stick saucepan, adding the onion, peppercorns, bay leaf and seasoning.
2 Heat gently and cover the pan. Simmer for 5 minutes. Turn off the heat and leave the milk mixture to stand with the lid on for a further 30 minutes or until you are ready to thicken and serve.
3 Mix the remaining milk with the cornflour and when almost ready to serve, strain the milk mixture, add the cornflour mixture and reheat slowly, stirring continuously until it comes to the boil. If it thickens too quickly, remove from the heat and stir very fast to mix well.
4 Add the chopped or dried parsley to taste, cook for 3–4 minutes and serve immediately.

SERVES 4
PER SERVING:
56 KCAL/0.2G FAT

300ml (½ pint) skimmed milk
1 onion, sliced
6 peppercorns
1 bay leaf
2 teaspoons cornflour
chopped fresh parsley or dried
    parsley to taste
salt and freshly ground black
    pepper

Spicy tomato and basil sauce

SERVES 4
PER SERVING:
16 KCAL/0.06G FAT

50g (2oz) onions, chopped
½ teaspoon chilli powder
1 × 115g (4oz) can plum
    tomatoes
2 teaspoons tomato purée
1 teaspoon caster sugar
¼ teaspoon oregano
1 tablespoon chopped fresh
    basil
salt and freshly ground black
    pepper

1 Dry-fry the chopped onions in a non-stick pan, using a little water if necessary to prevent burning.
2 When cooked, stir in the remaining ingredients and bring slowly to the boil, stirring continuously.
3 Simmer uncovered for 10–15 minutes so that the mixture reduces and becomes thicker. Taste for seasoning. This sauce may be frozen and stored for up to 2 months.

Red pepper sauce

SERVES 4
PER SERVING:
76 KCAL/1.9G FAT

3 red peppers
1 large onion, chopped
3 garlic cloves, finely chopped
300ml (½ pint) tomato passata
dash of Tabasco sauce
salt and freshly ground black
    pepper

This thick pepper sauce is ideal served with fish or meat and accompanies braised vegetables well. It can be thinned down with a little vegetable stock if required.

1 Preheat the oven to 200C, 400F, Gas Mark 6.
2 Prepare the peppers by slicing in half lengthways, remove the seeds and discard.
3 Place the peppers, onion and garlic in a non-stick roasting tin and season well with salt and pepper. Place in the oven for 30 minutes until the vegetables soften.
4 Remove from the oven and spoon into a food processor or liquidiser, add the passata and purée until smooth. Pass through a fine sieve to remove any stray seeds or skin. Reheat as required. Add Tabasco to taste.

Mushroom sauce

1. Heat all but 50ml (2fl oz) of the milk in a non-stick saucepan, adding the onion, peppercorns, bay leaf and salt and pepper.
2. Heat gently and cover the pan. Simmer for 5 minutes. Turn off the heat and leave the milk mixture to stand with the lid on for a further 30 minutes. Strain the milk through a fine sieve into a jug.
3. Rinse out the saucepan and then return the milk to it. Add the thyme, marjoram and chicken stock cube. Reheat to almost boiling.
4. Mix the cornflour and the remaining milk into a paste and slowly add this to the hot milk mixture.
5. Add the sliced mushrooms and gently heat until boiling, stirring continuously.
6. Continue stirring and cooking for a further 2 minutes. Taste to make sure there is sufficient seasoning and adjust as necessary.

SERVES 4
PER SERVING:
63 KCAL/0.6G FAT

300ml ($\frac{1}{2}$ pint) skimmed milk
1 onion, peeled and diced
6 peppercorns
1 bay leaf
$\frac{1}{2}$ teaspoon dried thyme
$\frac{1}{2}$ teaspoon dried marjoram
1 chicken stock cube
2 teaspoons cornflour
115g (4oz) button mushrooms, thinly sliced
salt and freshly ground black pepper

Creole sauce

SERVES 4
PER SERVING:
53 KCAL/0.5G FAT

1 large onion
1–2 garlic cloves or 1 teaspoon
    garlic paste
1 small green pepper
1 small red pepper
1–2 tablespoons lemon juice
1 teaspoon sugar
250g (10oz) tomato passata or
    canned tomatoes puréed
1 teaspoon French mustard
150ml (¼ pint) chicken stock if
    needed
1 tablespoon chopped parsley
salt and freshly ground black
    pepper

This sauce is good served with barbecued meats and fish.

1 Peel the onion and fresh garlic. Finely chop the onion and crush the garlic.
2 Remove the stalk, core, seeds and pith from the peppers and cut the flesh into small dice.
3 Place the onion, garlic, peppers, 1 tablespoon of lemon juice, sugar and the tomato passata or puréed tomatoes in a pan. Stir in the French mustard and season with salt and pepper.
4 Bring to the boil and simmer gently for 25–30 minutes until the onions and pepper are tender. If the sauce thickens too much during the cooking, add a little chicken stock while it is cooking and adjust the consistency and seasoning when the sauce is cooked.
5 Just before serving, add the parsley.

Bread sauce

1 Slowly bring the milk to the boil and add the chopped onion, cloves and bay leaf. Remove from the heat, cover the pan and leave to one side for 15–20 minutes to allow the flavours to infuse.

2 Remove the cloves and bay leaf, add the breadcrumbs and black pepper. Return to the heat, stir gently until boiling and season with salt and freshly ground black pepper.

3 Remove from the heat and place in a small covered serving dish (a small bowl covered with tin foil would work just as well). Keep warm until ready to serve.

SERVES 6
PER SERVING:
41 KCAL/0.19G FAT

300ml (½ pint) skimmed milk
1 small onion, chopped
3 cloves
1 bay leaf
6–8 tablespoons fresh
   breadcrumbs
salt and freshly ground black
   pepper

Brandy sauce

1 Heat all but 4 tablespoons of the milk with the almond essence until almost boiling and remove from the heat.

2 Mix the cornflour and remaining cold milk thoroughly and slowly pour it into the hot milk, stirring continuously until the mixture begins to thicken.

3 Return to the heat and bring to the boil. Continue to cook, stirring continuously. If it is too thin, mix some more cornflour with cold milk and add it slowly until you achieve the consistency of custard. Sweeten to taste.

4 Add the brandy a few drops at a time and stir well. Cover the serving jug and keep warm until ready to serve.

MAKES 600ML (1 PINT)
PER 600ML (1 PINT) OF SAUCE:
386 KCAL/0.8G FAT

600ml (1 pint) skimmed milk
3 drops almond essence
2 tablespoons cornflour
liquid artificial sweetener
3 tablespoons brandy

Minted fromage frais

SERVES 4
PER SERVING:
19 KCAL/0.1G FAT

fine zest and juice of 1 lemon
150ml (¼ pint) virtually fat free
fromage frais
1 tablespoon chopped fresh
mint
artificial sweetener to taste

This is delicious served with stewed apple or baked fruit.

1 Using the fine section of your grater, gently grate the outside zest from the lemon, taking care not to remove any of the white pith which may make the sauce bitter.
2 Mix with the remaining ingredients and pour into a sauce boat.

Orange or lemon sauce

SERVES 4
PER SERVING:
72 KCAL/0.1G FAT

300ml (½pint) skimmed milk
zest and juice from 2 oranges or
2 lemons
3 teaspoons arrowroot
artificial sweetener to taste
2 teaspoons orange liqueur
(optional)

1 In a non-stick saucepan heat the milk with the zest and juice from the 2 oranges or lemons to near boiling.
2 Mix the arrowroot with a little water to form a paste. Slowly stir into the hot milk and continue stirring to form a smooth sauce.
3 Sweeten to taste and add the liqueur if using.
4 Serve hot with pancakes or a baked apple.

Hot chilli sauce

Red chillies are the very hot ones, so do take care when using them. Start with just one chilli and add an extra one if necessary. When preparing them, make sure you do not touch your eyes, mouth or any tender skin with your hands. The seeds are also hot, so remove them if you want a much milder sauce. This is meant to be a thick sauce but you can dilute it with vegetable stock if you wish, although this will dilute the taste of the chillies. The sauce can be deep frozen.

1 Trim the chillies and remove the seeds if you wish. Chop the chillies finely.
2 Trim the spring onions and slice finely, or peel the onion if using and chop it finely.
3 Heat a non-stick pan, add the onions and some or all of the chopped chillies, according to preference. Cook gently until the onions are just soft but without colour.
4 Add 1 tablespoon of the lemon juice and the remainder of the ingredients. Season to taste with salt, sugar or artificial sweetener and extra lemon juice if required. At this stage you may also wish to add more chopped chilli.
5 Bring to the boil and simmer for 6–7 minutes. Taste again and adjust the seasoning if required.

SERVES 6
PER SERVING:
38 KCAL / 1.6G FAT

1–2 red chillies
2–3 spring onions or 1 small onion
1–2 tablespoons lemon juice
1 × 200g (7oz) can chopped tomatoes
2 tablespoons tomato purée
salt
1–2 teaspoons caster sugar or artificial sweetener to taste

Honey and orange sauce

SERVES 6
PER SERVING:
75 KCAL/0.5G FAT

1 large onion
1 garlic clove
150ml ($\frac{1}{4}$ pint) orange juice
2 tablespoons clear honey
3 tablespoons white wine
   vinegar
4–5 drops (a scant $\frac{1}{2}$ teaspoon)
   Tabasco sauce
2 teaspoons French mustard
1 sprig fresh rosemary
2–3 sprigs fresh thyme or $\frac{1}{2}$
   teaspoon dried thyme
salt and white pepper

This sauce is particularly good with poultry as well as lamb.

1 Peel the onion and garlic. Finely chop the onion and crush the garlic.
2 Mix all the ingredients together in a small pan and bring to the boil.
3 Simmer gently for 10 minutes or until the onion is tender. Serve hot.

Cranberry and port sauce

SERVES 6
PER SERVING:
33 KCAL/0G FAT

225g (8oz) cranberries
300ml ($\frac{1}{2}$ pint) cranberry juice
   drink
2 tablespoons port
artificial sweetener to taste
   (optional)

1 Place the cranberries in a saucepan. Add the cranberry juice drink. Bring to the boil, then simmer gently for about 5 minutes until soft. Push the mixture through a sieve to pureé it and return to the pan.
2 Stir in the port and heat through. Add a little artificial sweetener if desired.

Christmas the low-fat way

We tend to use this time of year as a celebration of food and festivity with the temptation to cast aside our regular eating pattern. Low-fat eating certainly does not mean we deny ourselves of some great traditional delights.

Making just a few minor adjustments such as reducing the fat content will make the food much lighter, allowing a little scope for that extra treat. Included are recipes for light starters, turkey and duck main courses with accompanying side dishes, wonderful vegetarian options and low-fat desserts suitable for all the family and guests alike.

Christmas would not be complete without a delicious Christmas pudding and a few mince pies for slim Santa and helpers.

Smoked salmon and lime pâté

SERVES 4
PER SERVING:
79 KCAL/1.8G FAT
PREPARATION TIME:
10 MINUTES

150g (5oz) fine sliced smoked salmon

juice of 2 limes

115g (4oz) virtually fat free fromage frais

50g (2oz) Quark (low-fat soft cheese)

1 teaspoon mixed peppercorns, crushed

This is deliciously light and tangy, making an ideal starter or simple lunch. Once refrigerated the pâté will keep for 5 days.

1 Flake the salmon into pieces and place into a food processor. Add the lime juice, fromage frais and Quark. Sprinkle a little pepper over and blend until smooth to form a soft pâté. Taste, adding a little more pepper if required, and blend again to combine.
2 Scrape the mixture out into a serving bowl or individual ramekins and refrigerate for 2 hours.
3 Serve with crusty bread and a few salad leaves as a starter or light lunch.

Seared scallops with carrot and pink ginger pickle

Scallops make an ideal starter, as they are quite fleshy in appearance yet light and delicate in both volume and flavour. Make the carrot salad in advance and store refrigerated until ready to serve.

1 Prepare the scallops by cleaning well under a cold running tap to remove any sand or grit. Pull away the small membrane attached to the side, being careful to keep the orange coral intact. Pat dry with kitchen towel and season well with salt and black pepper.
2 Using the coarse side of a grater, grate the carrot into a bowl and add the crushed coriander seed, peppercorns, ginger and vinegar. Season well, mixing the ingredients together. Mix in the fresh coriander and allow to sit for a minimum of 30 minutes.
3 Preheat a non-stick griddle pan with a little vegetable oil, then wipe out, using a good pad of kitchen paper.
4 Add the scallops to the pan and cook quickly for 1 minute on each side.
5 Arrange the carrot salad on a serving plate. Squeeze the lime over the scallops and remove from the heat. Place on top of the carrot, pouring the pan juices over.
6 Serve straight away with crusty bread.

SERVES 4
PER SERVING:
102 KCAL / 1.3G FAT
PREPARATION TIME:
20 MINUTES
SITTING TIME:
30 MINUTES
COOKING TIME:
10 MINUTES

12–16 large fresh scallops
225g (8oz) young carrots, peeled
½ teaspoon coriander seed, crushed
¼ teaspoon pink peppercorns
2 teaspoons Chinese pink ginger, finely sliced
1 tablespoon white wine or fruit vinegar
1 tablespoon chopped fresh coriander
salt and freshly ground black pepper
a little vegetable oil
1 lime, sliced in half

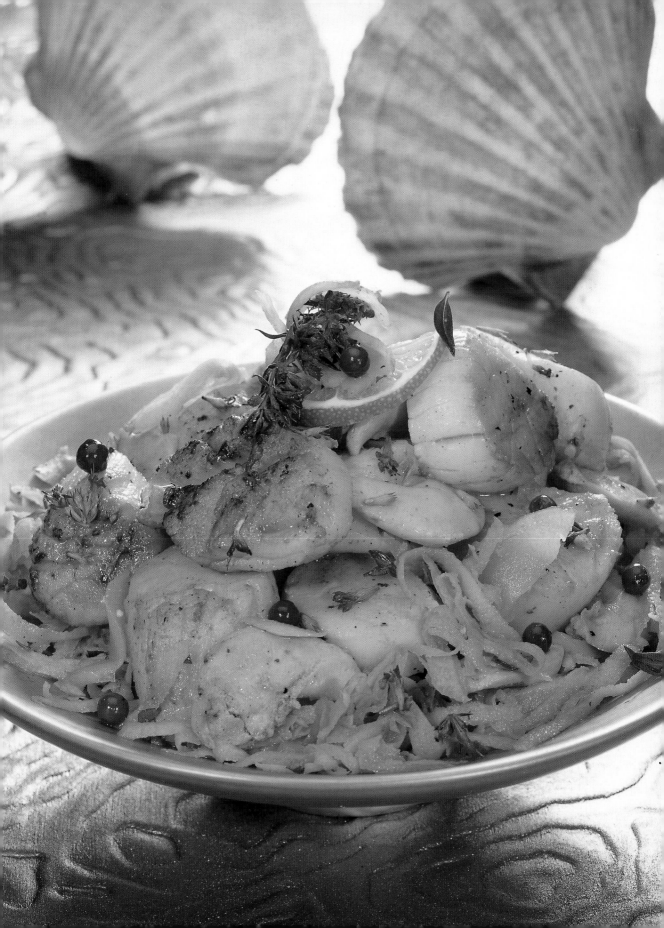

Roast turkey with chestnut stuffing and giblet gravy

1 Preheat the oven to 180C, 350F, Gas Mark 5.

2 Calculate the cooking time, allowing 15 minutes per 450g (1lb) plus an extra 20 minutes. Wash the turkey well in cold water and remove the giblets and any excess fat. Place the giblets, onion, bay leaves, and 2 sprigs of thyme in the centre of a large roasting tin and sit the turkey on top, preferably on its side.

3 Place the remaining thyme inside the turkey and season the outside generously with salt and black pepper. Pour 600ml (1 pint) of water around the outside of the turkey to prevent the base from burning, cover with foil and place in the oven.

4 Split the total cooking time into three, turning the bird onto its other side after one third of the cooking time and placing it breast side up for the final third. This will ensure even cooking.

5 While the turkey is cooking make the stuffing. Dry-fry the onion and garlic until the onion is soft. Add the breadcrumbs and herbs with a little black pepper. Mix in the stock, chestnuts and lemon and allow to stand for 10 minutes. Mould into golf ball-sized shapes and place on a non-stick baking tray.

6 Bake the stuffing in the oven for 20–25 minutes until brown and crisp.

7 Once the turkey is cooked, remove from the roasting tin and place on a serving dish. Keep it covered with foil and allow 30 minutes standing time for easier carving.

8 Drain the contents of the roasting tin into a saucepan. Remove the giblets and bay leaves and discard.

9 Use a ladle to skim off any fat from the top of the pan. Bring to the boil, adding more liquid if required, either chicken stock or water.

10 Slake the arrowroot with a little water and gradually stir into the gravy. Add a few drops of gravy browning if desired to colour the gravy. Adjust the consistency with more liquid or arrowroot.

11 Carve the turkey and serve with the chestnut stuffing, a selection of vegetables and the giblet gravy.

SERVES 10
PER SERVING:
APPROXIMATELY
200 KCAL / 4G FAT
PREPARATION TIME:
40 MINUTES
COOKING TIME:
3 1/2 HOURS

1 × 5.4kg (12lb) fresh turkey
1 large onion, diced
3 bay leaves
4–5 sprigs fresh thyme
pinch of sea salt
2–3 teaspoons arrowroot
a few drops gravy browning
freshly ground black pepper

for the stuffing
1 medium onion, finely chopped
1 garlic clove, crushed
115g (4oz) fresh breadcrumbs
1 tablespoon finely chopped fresh thyme
1 tablespoon chopped fresh parsley
300ml (1/2 pint) hot chicken stock
115g (4oz) peeled chestnuts, finely chopped
1 teaspoon finely grated lemon zest
black pepper to taste

Turkey pilaff

SERVES 4

PER SERVING:

355 KCAL/3.4G FAT

PREPARATION TIME:

15 MINUTES

COOKING TIME:

30 MINUTES

1 medium onion, finely chopped

2 garlic cloves, crushed

275g (10oz) [dry weight]
   basmati rice

750ml (1 $\frac{1}{4}$ pints) chicken stock

225g (8oz) cooked turkey

115g (4oz) chestnut mushrooms,
   sliced

4–5 sage leaves, finely chopped

3 bay leaves

salt and freshly ground black
   pepper

1 tablespoon finely chopped flat
   leaf parsley

Probably the simplest way of cooking rice and a great way to use up leftover turkey. For a vegetarian variation substitute the turkey with a few sundried tomatoes or canned artichoke hearts.

1 Preheat the oven to 190C, 375F, Gas Mark 5.

2 In a non-stick pan dry-fry the onion and garlic until soft. Add the rice and stock. Stir in the turkey, mushrooms, sage and bay leaves and season well with plenty of freshly ground black pepper.

3 Transfer to an ovenproof dish or casserole. Cover and place in the bottom of the oven for 25–30 minutes until the rice has absorbed all the stock.

4 Remove from the oven and serve sprinkled with chopped fresh parsley.

Braised duck with tangerine and cinnamon

This delicious duck recipe is perfect for Christmas entertaining, as all the preparation is done the day before. As it cooks it creates its own rich sauce full of aromatic flavours.

1 Prepare the duck by dividing into 4 portions. Using a sharp knife or heavy duty scissors, cut through the breastbone along the length of the bird then the backbone. Cut each piece in half again, cutting at an angle just under where the leg joint meets the carcass. Trim away the backbone and remove all of the skin, then place the duck in a large bowl.

2 Cut the tangerines in half and squeeze the juice over, adding the shells to the bowl. Season the duck well with sea salt and black pepper. Mix together the remaining ingredients and pour over the meat. Combine well, cover and refrigerate overnight.

3 Preheat the oven to 170C, 325F, Gas Mark 3.

4 Place the duck in a large casserole dish or non-stick pan, cover with foil and cook in the middle of the oven for 1½–2 hours until tender.

5 Remove from the oven and place the duck pieces on a serving plate. Pour the juices into a saucepan and adjust the consistency by adding a little more stock, or thicken by using 1 teaspoon of cornflour diluted with water.

6 Pour the sauce over the duck and serve garnished with the cooked tangerine shells.

SERVES 4
PER SERVING:
282 KCAL/11.4G FAT
PREPARATION TIME:
40 MINUTES
MARINATING TIME:
OVERNIGHT
COOKING TIME:
2 HOURS

1 × 2kg (4lb) duck
4 tangerines
300ml (½ pint) fresh apple juice
2 garlic cloves, crushed
2 cinnamon sticks
1 tablespoon fresh thyme
1 tablespoon Teriyaki sauce
150ml (¼ pint) chicken stock
2 tablespoons tomato purée
sea salt and freshly ground black pepper

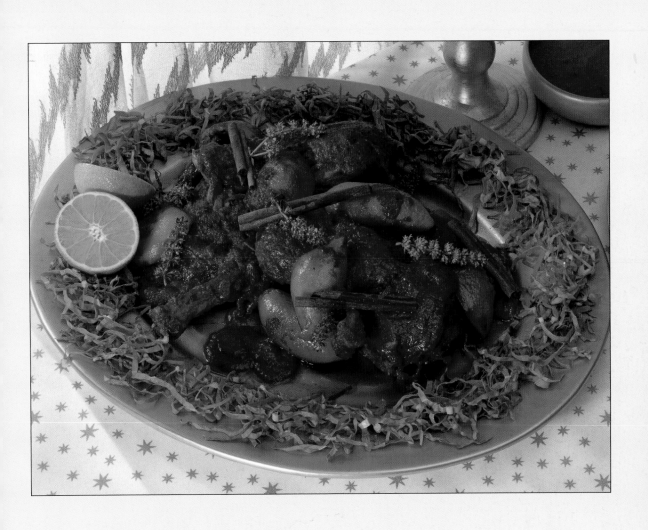

Marmalade basted gammon

A truly delicious way to prepare and serve Christmas ham. Star anise, its name deriving from its star-like shape, is popular in Asian cookery adding a sweet aniseed flavour throughout the dish. Use in moderation, as it can be bitter if used in excess.

1 Preheat the oven to 180C, 350F, Gas Mark 5.
2 Prepare the gammon by removing all the outer skin and fat with a sharp knife. Place in a large saucepan and cover with cold water.
3 Add the orange slices, anise, cloves, cinnamon and bay. Bring the pan to the boil, cover and simmer gently for 1 hour.
4 Transfer the gammon to an ovenproof dish, pouring some of the stock around to prevent it from sticking to the bottom of the dish. Coat the meat with the marmalade and bake in the oven, uncovered, for 20–25 minutes until golden brown. Sprinkle with sugar and return to the oven for 5–10 minutes until caramelised.
5 Allow to cool, then garnish with orange slices and whole cloves. Serve sliced cold with fruit chutney.

SERVES 8
PER SERVING:
420 KCAL / 12G FAT
PREPARATION TIME:
20 MINUTES
COOKING TIME:
1 HOUR 35 MINUTES

2kg (4¾lb) piece lean boiling bacon or gammon
3 oranges, sliced
2 star anise
6 whole cloves
2 cinnamon sticks
4 bay leaves
3 tablespoons Traditional thick-cut orange marmalade
2 teaspoons demerara sugar
1 orange to garnish
12 whole cloves to garnish

Lentil loaf with chestnut and herb stuffing

SERVES 6
PER SERVING:
256 KCAL / 6.4G FAT
PREPARATION TIME:
45 MINUTES
COOKING TIME:
40 MINUTES

225g (8oz) green lentils

1 vegetable stock cube

1 teaspoon sunflower oil

1 large onion, chopped

2 carrots, finely diced

115g (4oz) mushrooms, finely chopped

25g (1oz) chopped mixed nuts

75g (3oz) fresh white breadcrumbs

2 tablespoons chopped fresh parsley

2 tablespoons soy sauce

2 eggs, beaten

50g (2oz) herb stuffing mix

115g (4oz) canned chestnuts (drained weight)

This delicious vegetarian loaf can be served in place of the traditional turkey at the Christmas table.

1 Preheat the oven to 190C, 375F, Gas Mark 5.
2 Place the lentils in a large saucepan and cover with plenty of cold water. Add the stock cube and bring slowly to the boil, then boil rapidly for 10 minutes. Reduce the heat and simmer for 20–25 minutes until the lentils are tender. Drain.
3 Heat the oil in a large frying pan and fry the onion and carrots gently for 10 minutes until softened.
4 Add the mushrooms and cook for a further 3–4 minutes. Transfer to a large bowl and add the lentils, mixed nuts, breadcrumbs, parsley and soy sauce. Mix well. Add the beaten egg and mix again.
5 Very lightly grease the sides of a 1kg (2lb) loaf tin and line the base with baking parchment. Pile half the lentil mixture into the tin and press down well.
6 Mix the stuffing mix with 150ml ($\frac{1}{4}$ pint) cold water and allow to stand for a few moments. Chop the chestnuts and add to the stuffing.
7 Spoon a layer of stuffing on top of the lentil mixture in the tin. Cover with the remaining lentils and press down well. Cover with foil and bake in the oven for 40 minutes.
8 Allow to cool in the tin for 5 minutes before turning out onto a serving dish. Serve with cranberry sauce.

Roasted pepper and leek strudel

A great vegetarian dish packed full of flavour. It can be frozen cooked or uncooked. Vary the filling by using different combinations of cooked or roasted vegetables and serve with a simple spicy tomato sauce.

1 Preheat the oven to 200C, 400F, Gas Mark 6.
2 Cut the peppers in half, remove the seeds, and place face down in a non-stick baking tin. Roast in the top of the oven for 20–30 minutes until soft. Remove from the oven and place inside a plastic food bag. Seal the bag and leave to cool.
3 Preheat a non-stick frying pan and dry-fry the leeks with the thyme and garlic until soft, remove from the heat and stir in the basil, stock and passata.
4 Peel the cooled peppers, roughly chop and add to the leeks.
5 Separate the filo pastry sheets. Place one onto a non-stick baking tray and brush with the beaten egg. Continue adding the remaining sheets, brushing each layer with egg.
6 Spread the leek and pepper filling over the pastry, leaving a 2.5cm (1in) border around the edge. Fold in the 2 short sides and roll up like a Swiss roll. Brush the top with egg and bake in the oven for 8–10 minutes, until crisp and golden.
7 Make the sauce by heating all the ingredients in a small saucepan. Season with salt and pepper and serve piping hot.

SERVES 4
PER SERVING:
239 KCAL / 7.3G FAT
PREPARATION TIME:
40 MINUTES
COOKING TIME:
20 MINUTES

4 red peppers
4 baby leeks, sliced
a few sprigs fresh thyme
2 garlic cloves, sliced
handful of fresh basil leaves
1 teaspoon vegetable bouillon
    stock powder
2 tablespoons tomato passata
6 sheets filo pastry
    (30 × 20cm / 12 × 8in)
1 egg, beaten

for the sauce
300ml (1/2 pint) tomato passata
1 teaspoon ground cumin
1 teaspoon ground coriander
1 tablespoon chopped fresh
    coriander
1–2 teaspoons vegetable
    bouillon stock powder
salt and freshly ground black
    pepper

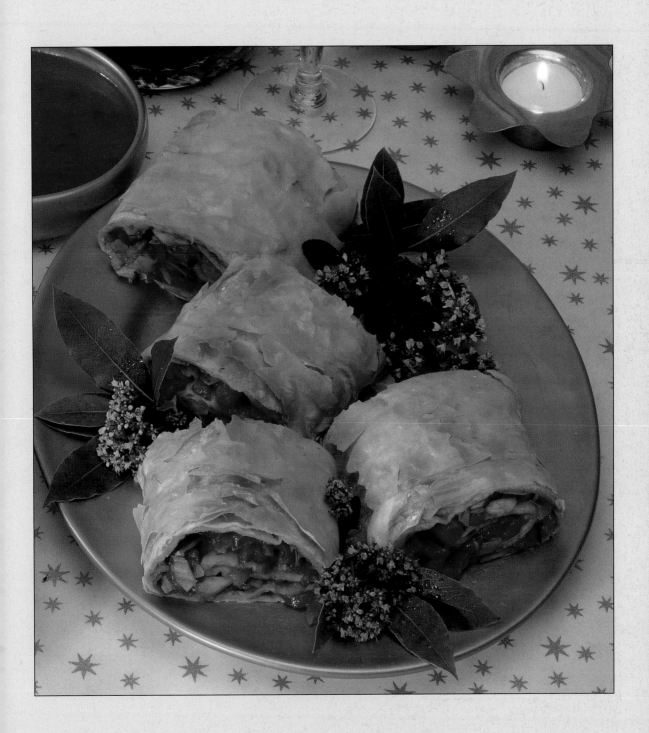

Caramelised onion bread sauce

Caramelising the onions adds a sweet concentrated flavour to this traditional sauce. The cloves add a little spice, but if you prefer, substitute with a little grated nutmeg.

1 In a non-stick frying pan, dry-fry the onions and garlic for 10–12 minutes until they start to colour and caramelise. Add the milk and remaining ingredients, stirring well to combine. Bring the sauce up to a gentle simmer and cook for 10 minutes to allow the flavours to develop.
2 Season well with salt and black pepper. Remove the cloves and bay leaves and pour the sauce into a serving dish.

SERVES 10
PER SERVING:
118 KCAL/0.7G FAT
PREPARATION TIME:
10 MINUTES
COOKING TIME:
30 MINUTES

4 medium onions, finely chopped
2 garlic cloves, crushed
300ml (½ pint) semi-skimmed milk
6–8 tablespoons fresh breadcrumbs
2 bay leaves
3 whole cloves
2 teaspoons vegetable bouillon stock powder
salt and freshly ground black pepper

Cranberry and orange relish

SERVES 10
PER SERVING:
66 KCAL/0.03G FAT
PREPARATION TIME:
10 MINUTES
COOKING TIME:
20 MINUTES

225g (8oz) fresh cranberries
115g (4oz) golden caster sugar
zest and juice of 2 oranges
1/2 teaspoon ground cinnamon
1 tablespoon ginger preserve
salt and freshly ground black
  pepper

A very useful relish to serve alongside hot or cold meats.
Refrigerated it will keep for up to 2 weeks.

1 Place the cranberries and sugar in a saucepan with 150ml
  (1/4 pint) water. Add the orange zest and juice, cinnamon and
  ginger preserve. Bring to the boil, reduce the heat and simmer
  gently for 15–20 minutes until the cranberries have split and
  the relish has reduced to a thick paste.
2 Season to taste with salt and black pepper, then allow to cool.
  Refrigerate until ready to use.

Brussels sprouts with pancetta and chestnuts

Adding a few extras to vegetables transforms them, providing texture and a contrast of flavours. For a vegetarian option substitute the pancetta with veggie bacon slices and cook in the same way.

1 Remove the loose outer leaves from the sprouts and make a small nick in the stalks. Cook in boiling water with the stock until just tender.

2 Meanwhile preheat a non-stick pan. Add the pancetta and cook quickly until it starts to crisp. Add the chestnuts and Brussels sprouts to the pan and continue cooking, mixing well.

3 Season well with salt, pepper and grated fresh nutmeg. Pile into a warm serving dish and serve.

SERVES 4
PER SERVING:
124 KCAL / 7.3G FAT
PREPARATION TIME:
20 MINUTES
COOKING TIME:
20 MINUTES

450g (1lb) Brussels sprouts
1 tablespoon vegetable stock
    bouillon or 1 stock cube
4 slices pancetta or smoked
    streaky bacon, finely chopped
115g (4oz) peeled and cooked
    chestnuts, chopped
grated fresh nutmeg
salt and freshly ground black
    pepper

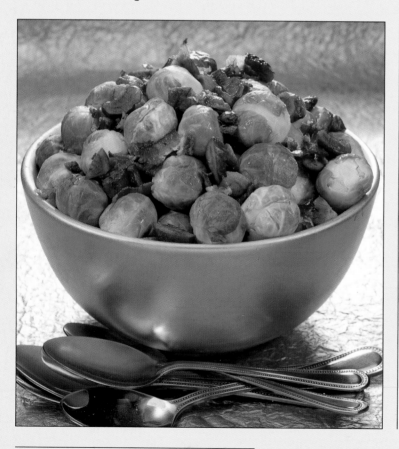

Roasted sweet potatoes with chilli glaze

SERVES 4
PER SERVING:
124 KCAL/0.5G FAT
PREPARATION TIME:
20 MINUTES
COOKING TIME:
55 MINUTES

450g (1lb) sweet potatoes
1 medium red onion, finely diced
2 tablespoons light soy sauce
1 teaspoon sea salt
1 red bullet chilli, seeded and
   finely chopped
1 garlic clove, crushed
2 tablespoons apple sauce
1 tablespoon chopped fresh
   parsley

Sweet potatoes make a good change from the regular, more common type. Naturally sweet, they complement strong meats such as duck or game. Delicious mashed with a little yogurt or fromage frais.

1 Preheat the oven to 200C, 400F, Gas Mark 6.
2 Wash, peel then rewash the potatoes and cut into 2.5cm (1in) pieces.
3 Boil in a pan of water for 5 minutes, then drain well. Place in the bottom of a non-stick baking tin with the red onion. Drizzle the soy sauce over and sprinkle with salt. Bake in the preheated oven for 20–25 minutes.
4 Remove from the oven. Combine the chilli, garlic and apple sauce and dot over the potatoes. Shake the pan well to coat, then return to the oven for 5 minutes. Sprinkle with parsley before serving.

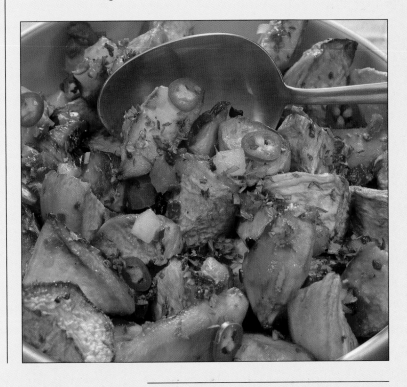

Creamed butternut squash

Butternut squash and carrot mashed together make a wonderful contrast of colours. This dish can be made in advance and reheated in the bottom of a moderate oven. Allow approximately 30 minutes.

1 Prepare the butternut squash by cutting in half with a large chopping knife. Scoop out the centre seeds and carefully peel away the outside skin. Chop the squash into bite-size pieces and place in a saucepan with the carrots. Cover with water.
2 Add the vegetable stock cube and mint and bring to the boil. Simmer gently for 15–20 minutes until the vegetables are tender.
3 Drain the vegetables well and return to the saucepan. Using a potato masher, mash until smooth. Stir in the fromage frais and season well with sea salt and black pepper. Pile into a serving dish and serve.

SERVES 4
PER SERVING:
120 KCAL/0.7G FAT
PREPARATION TIME:
15 MINUTES
COOKING TIME:
20 MINUTES

1 large butternut squash or 2 small
225g (8oz) carrots, chopped
1 vegetable stock cube
2–3 sprigs fresh mint
2 tablespoons virtually fat free fromage frais
sea salt
freshly ground black pepper

Braised spicy red cabbage

SERVES 8
PER SERVING:
62 KCAL / 0.4G FAT
PREPARATION TIME:
20 MINUTES
COOKING TIME:
1 1/2 HOURS

1 medium red cabbage

1 red onion, finely sliced

2 cooking apples, grated

5 juniper berries, crushed

pinch of red chilli flakes

75g (3oz) soft brown sugar

300ml (1/2 pint) red wine
    vinegar

150ml (1/4 pint) vegetable stock

salt and freshly ground black
    pepper

This flavoursome side dish can be made in advance and reheated in a low oven. It is especially good served cold alongside meats, fish and other buffet foods.

1 Preheat the oven to 150C, 300F, Gas Mark 2.
2 Cut the cabbage into quarters lengthways and remove the stalk. Finely shred the cabbage and place in a large mixing bowl.
3 Add the onion, apples, juniper and chilli, mixing all the ingredients together thoroughly and seasoning well with salt and black pepper.
4 Pile the mixture into a large ovenproof dish and sprinkle with brown sugar. Pour the vinegar and stock over and cover with greaseproof paper.
5 Bake in the bottom of the oven for 1–1 1/2 hours until soft.
6 Serve hot or cold as a vegetable accompaniment.

Banoffi whip

Treat yourself to a delicious creamy dessert that combines toffee custard and bananas. Don't make it too far in advance, as it may separate when stood for a while.

1 Using a fork, mash the bananas in a small bowl.
2 In a separate bowl mix together the sugar and custard powder with a little cold milk to form a smooth paste.
3 Heat the remaining milk in a saucepan with the rum, if using, until boiling, pour onto the custard powder and whisk well. Return to the pan and cook until the mixture starts to thicken. Remove from the heat, cover with food wrap and allow to cool.
4 Once cold, beat the yogurt into the custard mixture and sweeten to taste with a little sugar. Whisk the egg whites to stiff peaks and gently fold into the mixture. Spoon into individual glasses or 1 large bowl, dust with a little cocoa powder and decorate with fresh fruit.

SERVES 4
PER SERVING:
169 KCAL/0.8G FAT
PREPARATION TIME:
20 MINUTES
COOKING TIME:
15 MINUTES

2 bananas
1 tablespoon Muscovado sugar
1 tablespoon custard powder
250ml (8fl oz) skimmed milk
1 tablespoon rum (optional)
300g (11oz) low-fat Greek yogurt
2 egg whites
cocoa powder to dust

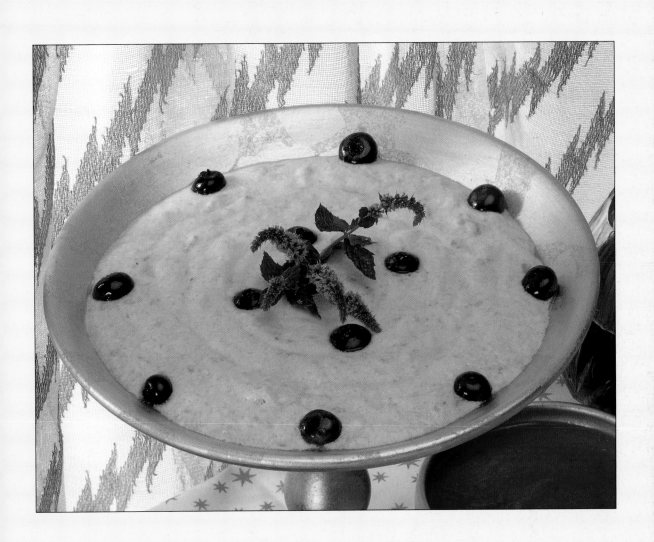

Fresh fruit flan

For a chocolate-flavoured base, substitute 25g (1oz) of flour with cocoa powder and add ½ teaspoon of baking powder. Choose fruits that will complement such as fresh orange or pears.

SERVES 6
PER SERVING:
146 KCAL/2.5G FAT
PREPARATION TIME:
20 MINUTES
COOKING TIME:
I HOUR

1 Preheat the oven to 180C, 350F, Gas Mark 4. Grease a 20cm (8in) non-stick flan case with a little vegetable oil then dust with caster sugar.

2 To make the sponge base, whisk together the eggs and sugar for several minutes until thick and pale in consistency. Using a metal spoon, fold in the sifted flour and then the vanilla. Pour into the prepared tin and level off with a knife. Bake in the oven for 20 minutes until golden brown.

3 Allow the sponge to cool, then using a serrated knife cut away a 1cm (½in) layer of sponge from the centre of the flan case. Using a metal spoon, scrape away the crumbs to leave a smooth surface.

4 Chop half the fruit into small dice and combine with the yogurt in a small bowl. Spoon the mixture into the centre of the sponge case and level, using a knife. Slice the remaining fruit and arrange on the top.

5 Heat the apricot jam in a small saucepan until liquid, then brush lightly over the fruit to glaze. Refrigerate until ready to serve.

6 Serve cold with virtually fat free fromage frais or 0% fat Greek yogurt.

2 eggs
75g (3oz) golden caster sugar
75g (3oz) self-raising flour, sifted
1 teaspoon vanilla essence
selection of fresh soft fruit approximately 225g (8oz) in weight, e.g. peaches, raspberries, apricots, kiwi
3 tablespoons Total 0% fat Greek yogurt
apricot jam to glaze

Compote of spiced fruits

SERVES 4
PER SERVING:
143 KCAL/0.3G FAT
PREPARATION TIME:
10 MINUTES
COOKING TIME:
15 MINUTES

225g (8oz) fresh dark plums
225g (8oz) fresh peaches
115g (4oz) soft dark sugar
150ml (¼ pint) cider vinegar
2 teaspoons coriander seeds
½ teaspoon allspice
zest and juice of 1 lemon
pinch of sea salt

Spiced fruits make an ideal accompaniment to cereals at breakfast or can be served warm as a dessert.

1 Cut the plums and peaches in half and remove the centre stones.
2 In a large saucepan dissolve the sugar in the cider vinegar over a low heat. Add the spices, lemon zest and juice and salt.
3 Add the fruits to the pan, cover and simmer gently for 15 minutes. Remove from the heat and allow to cool, still covered. Pour into a container and refrigerate until ready to use.
4 Serve cold or warmed with low-fat yogurt or low-fat fromage frais.

Christmas pudding soufflés

This is a much lighter version of this traditional celebratory pudding. Make sure the egg whites are whisked in a scrupulously clean bowl in order to achieve the maximum amount of volume.

1 Preheat the oven to 200C, 400F, Gas Mark 6.
2 Lightly grease 4 small ramekins with a little margarine, then dust lightly with caster sugar and set aside.
3 Place the fruit and other ingredients, except the brandy, in a small saucepan and simmer gently for 10–15 minutes until the fruit has reduced to a thick paste. Pour into a bowl, stir in the brandy and allow to cool.
4 In a clean bowl whisk the egg whites on full speed, adding only a pinch of sugar initially. Once the whites start to peak, gradually add the remaining sugar 1 dessertspoon at a time, allowing 10 seconds between each addition.
5 Place a teaspoon of fruit into the bottom of each ramekin, then gently fold the egg whites into the remaining fruit mixture. Pile into the ramekins, smoothing the top and sides with a palette knife. The mixture should stand about 5cm (2in) above the dishes.
6 Bake in the preheated oven for 5–6 minutes.
7 Serve immediately, as they will start to collapse as soon as they come out of the oven.

SERVES 4
PER SERVING:
260 KCAL/0.2G FAT
PREPARATION TIME:
20 MINUTES
COOKING TIME:
10 MINUTES

a little margarine
caster sugar to dust
1 small eating apple, cored, peeled and grated
50g (2oz) dried mixed fruit
25g (1oz) black cherries, pitted
1/4 teaspoon ground mixed spice
1/2 teaspoon grated orange zest
300ml (1/2 pint) fresh apple juice
1 tablespoon brandy

for the meringue
3 egg whites
175g (6oz) caster sugar
fresh fruit to decorate

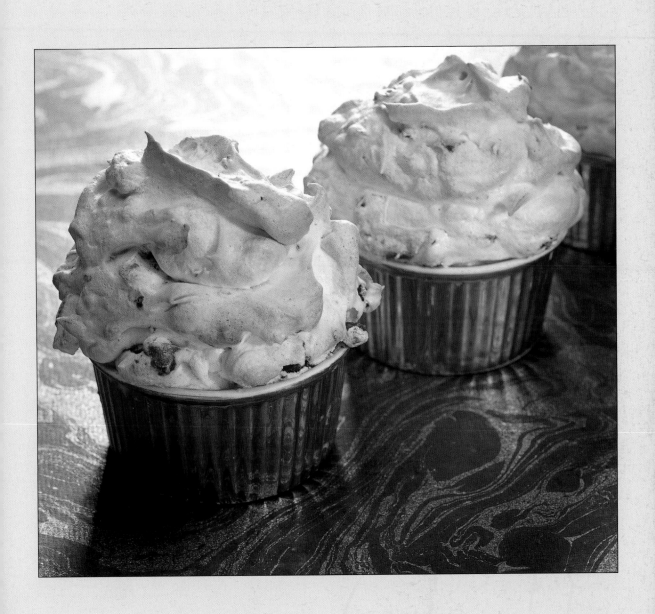

Spicy fat-free mincemeat

1 Place the dried fruit in a saucepan. Add the grated apple, mixed spice and cider.

2 Simmer for 20 minutes or until the mixture has formed a pulp and most of the liquid has evaporated.

3 Stir in the rum. Pack in sterilised jars and store in the refrigerator until required.

MAKES 1.5KG (3LB)
PER 1.5KG (3LB):
775 KCAL/1.1G FAT
PREPARATION TIME:
5 MINUTES
COOKING TIME:
20 MINUTES

225g (8oz) mixed dried fruit
150g (5oz) cooking apples,
   peeled and grated
$\frac{1}{2}$ teaspoon mixed spice
150ml ($\frac{1}{4}$ pint) sweet cider
2 teaspoons rum

Raspberry layer dessert

SERVES 4
PER SERVING:
240 KCAL/3G FAT
PREPARATION TIME :
20 MINUTES
COOKING TIME:
15 MINUTES

225g (8oz) low-fat sponge
   fingers
225g (8oz) fresh or frozen
   raspberries
2 egg whites
300ml ($\frac{1}{2}$ pint) Total 0% fat
   Greek yogurt
2 tablespoons icing sugar
2 tablespoons dry sherry
sprig of mint to decorate

A delicious refreshing dessert that is so simple to prepare. Try adding a little fruit liqueur in place of the sherry for a more luxurious flavour.

1 Place the sponge fingers in a food processor and reduce to fine crumbs or place in a plastic food bag and crush with a rolling pin.
2 Gently heat the raspberries, reserving a few for decoration, in a small saucepan over a low heat for 2–3 minutes until soft.
3 Whisk the egg whites until stiff then gradually fold in the yogurt and icing sugar.
4 Assemble the dessert in a glass dish in layers, first with the sponge finger crumbs sprinkled with sherry, then the raspberries and finally the yogurt mixture. Repeat, dusting the top with crumbs then place in the refrigerator until ready to serve.
5 Decorate with the reserved raspberries and a sprig of mint and serve chilled.

Filo pastry mince pies

1 Preheat the oven to 190C, 375F, Gas Mark 5.
2 Stack the filo pastry sheets on top of each other on the work surface. Using scissors, cut the stack into 6 square-shaped sections, so that you end up with 36 individual squares.
3 Take 6 non-stick patty tins. In each patty tin, place 4 individual pastry squares at slight angles to each other, brushing with beaten egg white in between each layer. Place a half tablespoonful of mincemeat in the centre of each pastry case.
4 Brush the remaining 12 pastry squares with egg white and scrunch them up to make crinkly toppings for the pies. Place 2 scrunched-up squares on top of each portion of mincemeat.
5 Bake in the oven for 10 minutes until the pastry is crisp and golden.
6 Just before serving, dust with a little icing sugar, if using.

MAKES 6 MINCE PIES
PER MINCE PIE:
144 KCAL/1.5G FAT
PREPARATION TIME:
20 MINUTES
COOKING TIME:
10 MINUTES

6 sheets filo pastry
    (12in × 8in/30cm × 20 cm)
1 egg white, beaten
3 tablespoons spicy fat-free
    mincemeat (see recipe, page
    260)
icing sugar to dust (optional)

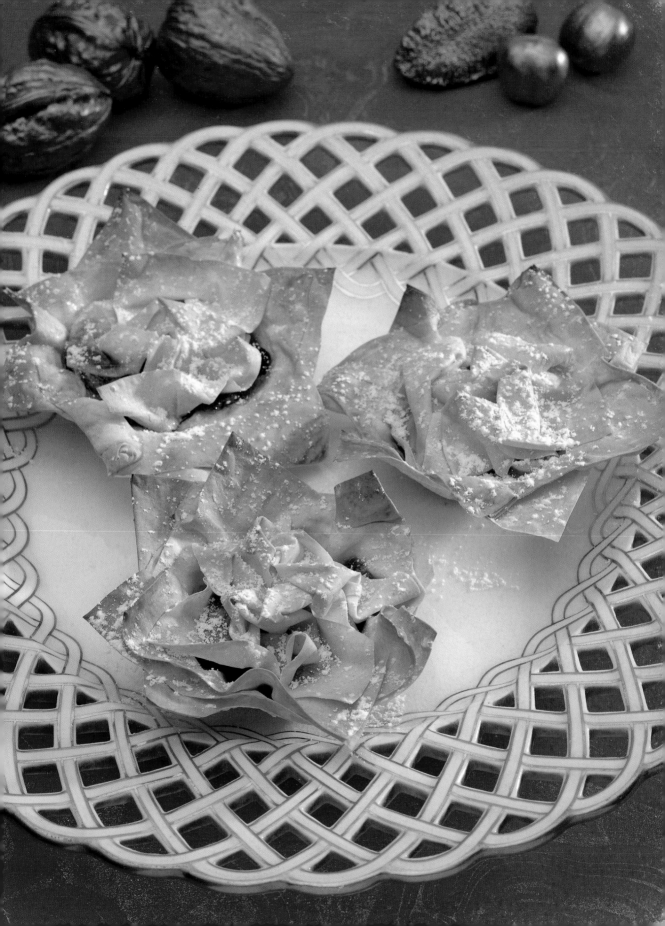

Tropical trifle

An alternative fruity dessert that makes use of unusual flavoursome fruits.

1 Make up the jelly according to the packet instructions, substituting 120ml (4fl oz) of the water with 2 glasses of sweet sherry.
2 Arrange the mango and pineapple in the bottom of a glass bowl. Cut 3 of the passion fruit in half and scoop out the seeds into the bowl. Pour the jelly over and refrigerate until set, preferably overnight.
3 When set, cover with the low-fat custard.
4 Place the vanilla pod onto a chopping board. Using the point of a sharp knife, split the pod down the centre lengthways. Run the blade of the knife along the pod, scraping out the vanilla seeds.
5 Add the seeds to the fromage frais and mix well. Spoon the fromage frais over the top of the custard and smooth with a knife. Decorate with seeds from the remaining passion fruit.

SERVES 4
PER SERVING:
290 KCAL/0.5G FAT
PREPARATION TIME:
10 MINUTES
COOKING TIME:
10 MINUTES

1 packet sugar-free jelly
2 sherry glasses sweet sherry
1 small mango, diced
1 small pineapple, cut into small
   pieces
4 passion fruit
1 × 425g (15oz) carton low-fat
   custard
1 vanilla pod
300g (10oz) virtually fat free
   fromage frais

Low-fat Christmas cake

MAKES APPROXIMATELY
20 SLICES
PER SLICE: 228 KCAL / 2.8G FAT
PREPARATION TIME:
30 MINUTES
COOKING TIME:
2–2 1/2 HOURS

225g (8oz) no pre-soak prunes,
   pitted
115g (4oz) cooking apple,
   grated
175g (6oz) dark Muscovado
   sugar
4 eggs, beaten,
zest of 1 lemon
zest of 1 orange
175g (6oz) self-raising flour,
   sifted
1 tablespoon mixed spice
50g (2oz) sunflower seeds
225g (8oz) currants
225g (8oz) sultanas
225g (8oz) raisins
115g (4oz) glacé cherries
120ml (4fl oz) brandy
2 tablespoons sieved apricot
   jam to glaze
12 glacé cherries to decorate

Cakes made without butter or margarine have a very different texture, probably best described as slightly chewy. They do, however, taste less greasy and more fruity. This cake benefits from being made at least one week in advance.

1 Preheat the oven to 170C, 325F, Gas Mark 3. Lightly grease and line a 20cm (8in), 7.5cm (3in) deep round tin with greaseproof paper.
2 In a large mixing bowl mash together the prunes and apple until smooth. Add the sugar then beat in the eggs a little at a time.
3 Mix in the zests, then carefully fold in the flour, mixed spice, sunflower seeds and dried fruit.
4 Gradually stir in the brandy and pour into the prepared tin. Arrange the cherries on the top and bake in the oven for 2–2 1/2 hours or until a metal skewer comes out clean once inserted in to the centre of the cake.
5 Allow to cool on a wire rack, then glaze by brushing with warmed apricot jam. Decorate with the glacé cherries.
6 Once cool, store in an airtight container.

Low-fat Christmas pudding

This is an old faithful recipe that tastes even better than the full-fat traditional pudding. No one will guess this is low fat – not even the greatest sceptic! You can deep-freeze the pudding, but do take care to thaw it thoroughly before reheating.

1 Soak the dried fruit in the brandy, rum or beer and leave overnight.
2 When ready to make the pudding, shake the cherries gently in the flour and then add the mixed spice, cinnamon, breadcrumbs, sugar and gravy browning.
3 Mix in the grated zest, apple and carrot, together with the lemon juice. Add the soaked fruit.
4 Beat the eggs with the milk and molasses and slowly add to the mixture, stirring well. Mix together gently and thoroughly.
5 Place in a 1.2 litre (2 pint) ovenproof basin. If you are going to microwave the pudding, place an upturned plate over the basin and microwave on high for 5 minutes. Leave to stand for 5 minutes, then microwave for a further 5 minutes. If steaming the pudding, cover with foil or a pudding cloth, and then steam gently for 3 hours (this makes a moister pudding).
6 After cooking, allow the pudding to cool and then wrap in aluminium foil and leave in a cool, dry place until required.
7 Before reheating, pierce the pudding several times with a fork and pour some more rum or brandy over the top. Steam for 1–2 hours or microwave on high for 10 minutes.
8 Serve with brandy sauce (see page 232).

SERVES 10
PER SERVING:
280 KCAL/2.5G FAT
SOAKING TIME:
12 HOURS
PREPARATION TIME:
20 MINUTES
COOKING TIME:
MICROWAVING: 15–20 MINUTES
STEAMING: 5 HOURS

75g (3oz) currants
75g (3oz) sultanas
115g (4oz) raisins
4 tablespoons brandy, rum or beer
75g (3oz) glacé cherries, halved
75g (3oz) plain or self-raising flour
1 teaspoon mixed spice
1/2 teaspoon ground cinnamon
50g (2oz) fresh breadcrumbs
50g (2oz) Muscovado or caster sugar
2 teaspoons gravy browning
grated zest of 1/2 lemon
grated zest of 1/2 orange
115g (4oz) grated apple
115g (4oz) finely grated carrot
1 tablespoon lemon juice
2 eggs
4 tablespoons skimmed milk
2 tablespoons molasses or cane sugar syrup
4 tablespoons rum or brandy for reheating

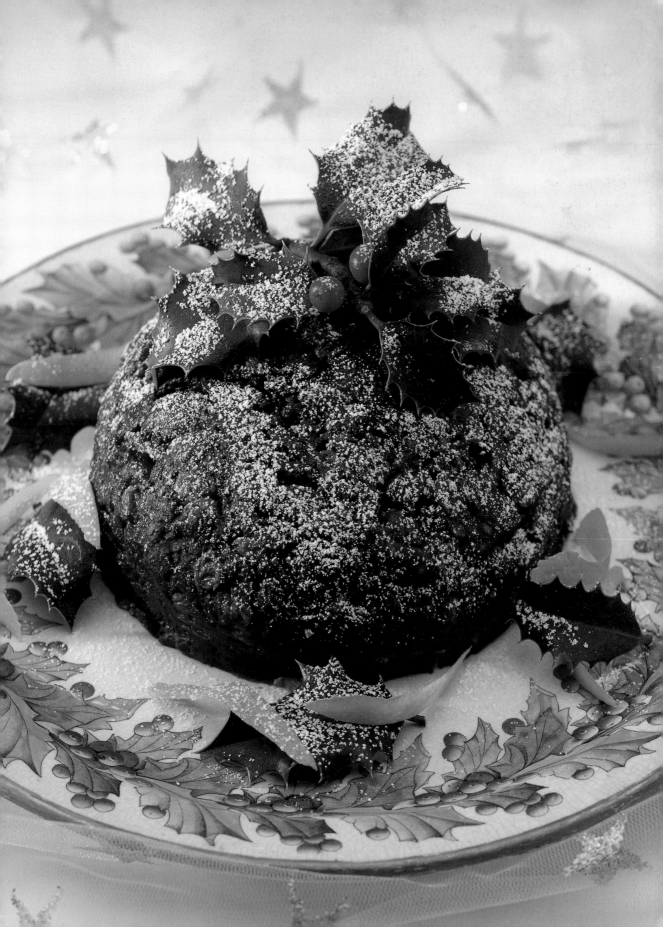

Index